easy
sexy
raw

ALSO BY CAROL ALT

Eating in the Raw:
A Beginner's Guide to
Getting Slimmer, Feeling
Healthier, and Looking
Younger the Raw-Food Way

The Raw 50: 10 Amazing
Breakfasts, Lunches, Dinners,
Snacks, and Drinks for Your
Raw Food Lifestyle

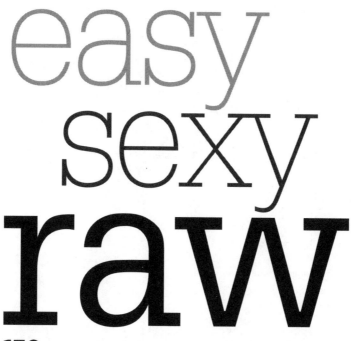

easy
sexy
raw

130 RAW FOOD RECIPES, TOOLS, AND TIPS
TO MAKE YOU FEEL GORGEOUS AND SATISFIED

carol alt

with leda scheintaub

clarkson potter/publishers
new york

Copyright © 2012 by Altron II, Inc.
Photographs copyright © 2012 by Usha Menard

Published in the United States by Clarkson Potter/Publishers, an imprint of
the Crown Publishing Group, a division of Random House, Inc., New York.
www.crownpublishing.com
www.clarksonpotter.com

CLARKSON POTTER is a trademark and POTTER with colophon is a
registered trademark of Random House, Inc.

Library of Congress Cataloging-in-Publication Data
Alt, Carol
    Easy sexy raw / Carol Alt.—1st ed.
        p.   cm.
    1. Raw foods.   2. Raw food diet—Recipes.   3. Cookbooks   I. Title.
    TX392.A427   2012
    613.2'65—dc23   2011025696

ISBN 978-0-307-88869-3
eISBN 978-0-307-88870-9

Printed in the United States of America

Book design and cover design by Rae Ann Spitzenberger
Book and cover photography by Usha Menard

10 9 8 7 6 5 4 3 2 1

First Edition

Big differences can come
from little changes.

contents

the recipes

foreword

BY NICHOLAS J. GONZALEZ, M.D.

IT HAS NOW BEEN MORE THAN SEVEN YEARS since Carol's first book, *Eating in the Raw*, appeared to wide acclaim, and more than three years since the second, *The Raw 50*, was published. Both books passionately and wisely spoke about how the world is in need of healthy eating—with an emphasis on whole raw foods—and about how the potential for great health lies within our grasp.

We need such guidance more than ever before, for the statistics would seem to show that our health in America isn't very good and that it continues to deteriorate, with heart disease, cancer, and other major diseases on the rise. Despite the advances of modern drug-based, high-tech medicine, disease is around us and it's clear that it can wreak havoc in our lives. But there is good news: vibrant lasting health is not some mythic ideal but a question of choice—particularly choice regarding the food we eat.

In the foreword to Carol's last book, I touched on the classic text *Nutrition and Physical Degeneration*, written by the dentist Weston Price and first published in 1945, and which is a major influence on my practice. Though this text is well known and widely read within the alternative medical world, in the academic medical universe the book is unknown and typically never read. How does that figure into the world of eating raw? Read on and I'll explain.

For some seven years beginning in the 1920s, Dr. Price traveled the world studying isolated groups of humans who were still following a way of life largely untouched by Western industrialization. Price's journey took him from the Arctic of the Eskimos, to the high Andes of the Inca descendents, to the African savannah of the Masai, to the high mountain valleys of Swiss Alpine herders, to Polynesia and its fisherman culture, and just about everywhere else in between. Price focused his attention on the diet and the health of the people living according to centuries-old wisdom about food and eating. Then he investigated the dietary habits and health of those people in each area who had migrated to regional towns and adopted a more Westernized lifestyle and eating pattern, consisting primarily of canned, processed, refined, overcooked, and highly sweetened foodstuffs shipped from long distances. He compared the incidence of various diseases, such as cancer, dental caries, and tuberculosis among those living a traditional life to those eating "Western."

Wherever Dr. Price journeyed, tribes and communities of humans who still followed a traditional locally and freshly obtained, whole, unprocessed, unrefined, often largely raw foods diet enjoyed superb and enduring good health. These peoples seemed remarkably immune not only to infectious diseases such as tuberculosis, but also to degenerative illnesses already reaching epidemic and near-epidemic proportions in Price's day, such as arthritis, cancer, dental disease, diabetes, heart disease, and stroke.

Among those who had migrated from their traditional communities, Price recorded a drastic change in diet—and ultimately a catastrophic deterioration in their health. These folks no longer consumed the wholesome fruits and foods from the land but the fruits and foods of modern industry, heavily cooked and refined. Those who might have only recently abandoned the traditions of their ancestors still enjoyed fairly good health, though not as vibrant or as disease-free as their cohorts who still lived and ate as their ancestors had. But among the offspring of the citified migrants, living from infancy on the industrialized foods favored by their parents, Price documented an extraordinary surge in various illnesses, an avalanche of arthritis, cancer, dental disease, heart disease, and infectious disease such as tuberculosis. Price believed only the industrialized diet could explain this profound and rapid fall from good health.

In Price's worldview, appropriate diet and nutrition provide us with the tools we need to allow for healthy and long lives, free of the majority of diseases we fear so much in the civilized West. Far from some inevitable process, these diseases largely develop because of our own doing, as we live and eat indifferent to cultural traditions, enamored of a technology and industrialized agriculture that may ultimately be more of a problem for us than a solution.

Of course, now more than sixty years have passed since the publication of Price's book, and most of the traditional cultures he studied have long vanished, and many people ask if there is a way his findings can be incorporated into their lives. The answer is a resounding yes, and books such as this one and Carol's first two certainly provide us with a road map to start on the journey.

Price noted that we humans thrived on a variety of diets, from all meat (the Eskimos) to more plant based (the Polynesians), though the majority were somewhere in between. So forget the dictates of any expert who says he or she has discovered the "one perfect diet" for all of us. There is no such thing; there are many perfect diets.

But in our genetically mixed modern society, how do we translate this information into a practical way of healthy eating for our modern lives? In our office we have specialized tests that help us with great accuracy sort through the confusion rampant in the nutritional world regarding the so-called right diet, but I understand that such tests are not widely available. The good news is that there are very simple ways of guiding one toward the proper diet—and believe it or not, one's basic food preferences can point us in the right direction. So if you aren't certain of your ancestry or your ancestry is mixed, go by what healthy foods you are drawn to (think green vegetables and protein rather than empty foods like coffee and sugar, which might draw you in but soon after result in a crash) and see how you feel when you eat them. While nutrition is indeed a science, I find that returning to our dietary instincts is a commonsense way of working toward an optimum individual diet.

For example, I find that people who by genetics and ancestry should be eating a meat-based diet invariably love meat, and they love fat—the more fat the better. They couldn't care less if they never ate another salad and tend not to care for fruit. They don't tolerate grains well but enjoy legumes, root vegetables, squash, cruciferous vegetables like broccoli and Brussels sprouts, and fermented vegetables like sauerkraut. We often suggest that they consider cooking their meat as little as possible—even indulging in steak tartare if they like.

In my practice, even though my colleague Dr. Linda Isaacs and I prescribe for our "carnivore patients," as we call them, lots of fatty meat— an anathema to more conventional doctors—such people metabolize saturated fat and cholesterol very efficiently; in fact they need such nutrients to make energy on a cellular level, and never, in my experience, develop atherosclerosis and heart disease. In contrast, they cannot efficiently use carbohydrates, which in them tends to provoke hypoglycemia and eventually insulin resistance and diabetes. (An interesting fact: The traditional Eskimo, or Inuit, ate a fair amount of their fatty meat raw—for them raw blubber and fermented fatty fish like salmon were both special treats containing many important enzymes— yet they never developed heart disease, as Western researchers have confirmed.) As Carol's books include information on incorporating animal products into the raw diet, I feel she is filling a gap that most vegan raw food books on the market have left.

On the other hand, our vegetarian patients tend to gag at the thought of pot roast or fatty meats, and do just fine with a salad and some fruit for lunch—hypoglycemia is not something they tend to experience, even after eating a light plant-based, high-fruit meal. They like and thrive on raw vegetables, fresh vegetable juices, and lots and lots of fruit—the more the better. We find as did Price that no humans do well long term on a purely plant-based diet, so even for our "vegetarian" patients we allow some limited animal protein, the amount varying from person to person. Overall, such people do best with about 70 to 80 percent or more of their food in the raw state—and despite the current fear of grains and grain products such as bread in the alternative medical world, our "plant eaters" generally tolerate these foods well, though they should be organic and preferably sprouted, a process, as Carol has shown so eloquently, that increases nutrition and reduces allergic reactions.

Our "balanced metabolizers," as we call them, fall somewhere in between the "carnivores" and "vegetarians." They tend to crave and do best with a variety of food sources, of both plant and animal origin. They thrive at a buffet where they can pick and choose different foods, including fruits, vegetables, nuts, seeds, grain products, eggs, dairy, fish, poultry, and red meat. They also do well with about 50-percent raw, 50-percent cooked, and tend to go through periods when they might crave more raw, or less raw, and periods when they might desire more plant than animal foods, or vice versa.

Not what you were expecting from a foreword to a book on raw foods? Well, as Carol stresses throughout her book, the amount of raw that is right for you is an individual decision, based on a variety of factors. Carol's book will serve you wherever you are with raw, whatever type of eater you are. So you should favor clean, unprocessed food while finding the raw point that feels most comfortable for you. Eat hearty, eat well—and bask in the vibrant health that it brings. With the wonderful recipes that Carol has shared here, that won't be hard to do!

introduction

I AM GUESSING THAT THE TITLE OF THIS BOOK compelled you to pick it up. I hoped it would! And I am sure that the word "sexy" was a major factor in your decision. But you may be wondering how food—especially raw food—could be sexy.

My answer? Anyone who saw the movie *9½ Weeks* cannot argue that food isn't sensual: Those were raw strawberries that Mickey Rourke fed Kim Basinger in that memorable, steamy kitchen floor scene. And then the honey, sticky and dripping everywhere . . . need I go on?

Yes, food can be very sexy. But health, glorious health, is the "sexy" I am thinking of. The energy and glow that come with health are beyond compare and cannot be manufactured.

On the other hand, I cannot think of anything less sexy than sickness. Hospitals and blood tests and pills with side effects are so not sexy. I always say to my friends and family that once you have lost your health, no matter how many Mercedes you have in your driveway, you will not be happy or have a sense of well-being and peace. If sickness was hanging over your head, you would sell anything, do anything, to get your health back. I know, because I have been there.

This book is going to make keeping or regaining your health fun—by making raw foods a part of your life. Yes,

fun! Once you see how easy and no-fuss my approach is and the large variety of foods you have to choose from, turning your meals raw will be something to look forward to.

I haven't had a cold in the fifteen years that I've been raw. Nor a headache. Ditto for the flu, sinus infections, stomachaches, heartburn, or cramps—I could go on and on. Yet the only thing I did was to change my food habits. I went raw, and have eaten raw foods almost exclusively for the last fifteen years. And when I fall off raw—yes, I am human—I start to see those ugly problems rear their heads.

So I take the hint and go right back on raw.

The good news: While there are misconceptions of what "normal" health is, true good health is in fact possible. When I started getting heartburn and headaches at age twenty-seven, everyone told me that it was normal. When I started to get fine lines and wrinkles, I was told "that is just part of aging; get used to it." Well, if it is, then I pose this question: How come fifteen years later, I have reversed these issues?

Going raw has made the difference between sickness and health for me, and I am not the only one who has seen amazing, wonderful things happen to her body from eating this way. There are now many books on raw foods, so there must be something to it! Over the years I have been seeing more and more people transition to this way of life. And I do say "way of life" because this is not a diet per se.

The raw way of eating will affect your whole life. When my friend Steven Cantor told me about how eating raw helped his girlfriend reverse her cancer, he suggested that I speak with the doctor who helped her, Dr. Timothy Brantley. He told me I would look at food differently. I then changed what I ate and my life changed, too. He was so right—I now look at raw food as life-saving, and that is how I stay so faithful to eating raw!

If you are asking me if raw food is a miracle, then I will answer you that for me it was. It was such a huge miracle—

prolonging my life and my career, creating a better, pain-free life, anti-aging me, and giving me freedom and control over my health—that I had to pass on the secret. But first I urge you to find a doctor who understands raw and can monitor you and your body's acceptance of raw.

Believe me, I tried so many of the diets out there that I starved myself right into poor health. And with the state of our health, it is obvious to me that others are doing the same thing I was doing. So I am here to offer hope and help.

When I talk at health conventions, I say that food is the most powerful drug we have. And I should know, I saved my own life with it—or so my doctor told me.

raw: before and after

I know what you're thinking: You're Carol Alt, you're genetically blessed, but what about me? Well, I may be model-tall, but believe me, I'm not naturally model-thin. In fact, my life before going raw was fairly miserable. My diet was so bad for so long that my health and weight were spiraling out of control. I had horrible blood sugar swings. And I'm not kidding, I'd literally gain weight if I ate one baked potato. I had to starve myself to maintain my weight, and in starving myself, I got the health issues that went along with not properly nourishing the body. General malaise, heartburn, sinus infections, stomach acid, headaches, chronic tiredness, colds, flu, asthma, and worse—I had them all. Genetically blessed? I wish. It was a nightmare before I went raw.

As a model I wouldn't eat all day until I "rewarded" myself with a brownie sundae—obviously I was sugar addicted.

It was such a hardship to sit at dinners where I couldn't eat anything because I thought that salads were "fattening"; even olive oil seemed fattening. (Cooked olive oil is more fattening than cold-pressed olive oil eaten in the right amount—but who knew?) I would pick at lunch in the studio, but not eat dinner. I started becoming antisocial because it was just easier not to be around food or people eating.

Even when I thought I was eating the right things, I wasn't getting the right results. When I wasn't doing the starving all day–brownie sundae at night routine, I would follow a strict regimen of what I believed was healthy food in controlled portions. I subsisted on boring foods that I assumed I was supposed to eat, like pasta or boiled chicken breast with steamed vegetables or the above-mentioned baked potato. While this was a step up from starving myself, these sparse meals would leave me distinctly unsatisfied.

Like many of you, I grew up in the age of convenience foods; canned food, TV dinners, and frozen pizza were the norm at our table. I didn't even realize that broccoli was green until I started modeling—I always knew it as something gray and mushy and a little scary. I'd never seen a crudité in my life, and I didn't even know what raw fish looked like; my mother would broil it until it was tough like the leather in your shoes. No offense to Mom. She did make the best spaghetti, and I used to stand by the pot and dip bagels in the sauce as it was cooking. I thought steak was tough and tasteless, so I would dress it with bottled Caesar dressing; I didn't know the problem was that it was always overcooked until it was dry and stiff. When I was a teenager, store-bought ice cream was my afternoon treat and, alas, I worked at a bakery—need I say more about my diet growing up?

what happened to our food?

I love the people who challenge me with "My grandmother lived until ninety, smoking Camel no-filters and drinking scotch."

My response? Genetics aside, the generations before ours had something we didn't have—genuinely clean, unprocessed food, which gave their bodies a natural advantage. The foods were closer to nature, with more of their enzymes, vitamins, and minerals intact.

The fundamental change to our diets is very important to understand. Before mass pasteurization of milk, the milkman delivered life-promoting enzymes and nutrients, and children built up their immunity with raw milk, butter, and cheese. Now we go to the supermarket to buy milk so devoid of life that it has to be fortified, and the added vitamins aren't the same as the ones we should be getting naturally.

Our generation is one big science experiment, and it is getting worse: We are now irradiating food and genetically modifying it. We have been playing God with our food, and we have no idea what the consequences are—but we are beginning to get a good idea.

Youth can more or less keep us running for a while, but once that nutritional reserve runs out, all that dead food will catch up to us; it's just a matter of when. For me, I could see a distinct difference in my health between the ages of twenty-two and thirty-two. I was headed on a sharp downhill ride, and I could feel it! When I was twenty-two, I didn't take a pill. I had energy to burn. When I was thirty-two, there was a pill for my sinuses, a pill for my headaches, a pill for my indigestion, a pill to sleep. Then coffee to wake myself up! I thought to myself, "If this is me at thirty-two, what will I be like at forty? Or fifty?" (Yikes! Fifty comes fast!) I didn't even want to think about it. I could see the road I was heading down and decided to make a sharp U-turn.

my u-turn: talking to dr. timothy brantley

I took my friend Steve Cantor's advice and called Dr. Timothy Brantley. He was unlike any doctor I had ever spoken to before. He did not ask me what my problems were or how I was feeling. He asked me, "What do you eat?" Strange question, I thought. I replied that I started my day with coffee, and I ate pasta, bread, and worse. He laughed and mentioned that he would be surprised if I didn't have sinus infections, headaches, general tiredness, malaise, and indigestion. I thought, "Holy cow, he just assessed my main problems."

It was right then and there that I decided to give up the insanity. I decided to try something new and completely different. What Dr. Brantley taught me changed my life. He taught me about feeding my body to the point where it heals itself, stays thin, and doesn't need any medications. He taught me about eating raw. At thirty-four, I had won the jackpot. My life was turned around and I could eat everything—oil on my fish, butter, or cream—as long as these foods were made with cold-pressed, raw, and unpasteurized products. Dr. Brantley gave me a new lease on my life, and ever since then it has been my mission to pay it forward.

the transition

Everyone transitions to raw in his or her own way—I went cold turkey, but then again, not everyone is as type A as I am. Gradual and steady may seem boring, but it just might be the best way for you to ease yourself in. Keeping some of the healthier cooked food choices in your diet for a while may ensure that you don't cleanse too quickly and help to minimize detox symptoms. And when it's not all or nothing, there's no guilt, and you can't "fall off," can you?

nothing happens all of a sudden

Everything we do to the body is cumulative, according to Dr. Brantley. It is amazing how many times I hear people use the words "all of a sudden." All of a sudden I got wrinkles, all of a sudden I looked in the mirror and saw my mother/father. All of a sudden I had cancer. But these things don't happen all of a sudden. Our health or lack of it is not something that happens overnight.

That said, my diet was so bad and my body so depleted that I was really ready for the switch. Detoxing was a step up for me. I started to get results within three days. You heard me, three days! After three days, my sinus infections went away. After a month, my energy picked up and my bloat went away, as did the symptoms my previous doctor missed. People started reacting differently to me; I was walking around with a huge grin on my face—I couldn't help it. The weird thing is that I did not even realize how bad I had been feeling until I started to feel good!

Great things began to happen to me because I was radiating positive energy. My body realized it was getting good food, and it was now calling for it big time. I started eating 100 percent raw foods like a crazy woman for the first month—without gaining weight! My body was cleaning and healing itself while stocking up on minerals and nutrients. Then suddenly my body said, "Okay, Carol, I get it, you're going to feed me real food as a rule now." I finally was nourished to the point that my eating slowed down.

Now that I'm eating raw, instead of getting stressed out about food, I'm happy to eat. I never feel guilty about what I eat. I never get that fat thigh–big butt feeling when I get up from the table. And I never need to pick. I had a big realization: Food is not entertainment, it is not a luxury. It is a necessity. But it should not control me; I should control it, and I should make that necessity enjoyable along the way!

So if I can save one person from the road I traveled and help them to become healthy and happy—and feed them marvelous food along the way— it's all worth it.

what is raw food?

There are some key principles to going raw, and back when I started out there were few resources out there to guide us raw pioneers. The raw lifestyle was as fringe then as it is fashionable now—there wasn't a raw olive or a raw pickle to be had, and I made all my own food. And of course there were many misconceptions. (I'll share with you one rule of thumb that helped me: If you have to ask, then it's probably cooked. Remembering this makes things much, much easier.)

Raw food is, simply put, food in its natural, unprocessed, and uncooked state. It can be heated, but not really above the magic temperature of 115°F. (For anyone who wants to get more into it, I have included a section called In My Opinion . . . What It Means to Be Raw [page 245], that tells you more about what happens to your food when it is cooked.)

the more raw the better

As this is a raw foods book, obviously I am encouraging you to go raw! But let me be clear: Even if you don't become a raw foodist, the more raw food you add to your diet, the more benefits you will see. (And my recipes are by no means a mere substitution for cooked food; they are, plain and simple, great food that strict raw foodists, dabblers, and everyone in between can enjoy!) You don't have to be 100 percent raw to see changes in your health; just know that whenever you eat your food raw, you're taking a step toward a healthier and more nourished you.

"what do you eat? carrots?"

I decided to write my first book, *Eating in the Raw* (2004), because people were always asking me what I ate. More times than not they guessed carrots! I am not sure why carrots seem to signify health food or raw food (and feature in so many jokes about raw), but I wrote the book to let people know that there was way more to raw foods than sprouts and crunchy vegetables. I can eat tiramisu, that wonderfully creamy Italian dessert, for example, as long as it is raw. Or ice cream, or pie even, when they are raw.

In this book I will explain and demystify what raw means, and I will share what I have learned so that you can transition to eating raw, or if not totally raw, then at least healthier. And I will even teach you how to make raw cookies. (Hint: It's just a matter of dehydrating them. See pages 72 and 209.)

who me, vegan? nah!

I'd like to set straight a small but important detail up front: This book is not vegan. Yes, that's right. There are plenty of recipes that could be called vegan, but there are also recipes with raw dairy, raw fish, and raw meat. Call me blasphemous (go ahead—I've been called worse), but I don't see how raw equals vegan. Eating vegan is a personal choice, and maybe a choice that you make with your doctor, but it's not intrinsic to being raw. Eating raw means eating food that is not cooked. Simple! So if you don't eat pasteurized dairy or canned, jarred, or prepared foods, then you've got a head start on becoming a raw foodist. I enjoy raw milk, raw-milk cheeses, kefir, sashimi, and more—that is, in moderation. Fish a couple of times a week, and a sprinkle of raw-milk cheese on a salad here and there are just the right amount of animal products to balance out my diet. My philosophy is to eat what you like as long as it's prepared correctly—in other words, raw—and I must say that most people I meet like having a little dairy, meat, or fish in their diets.

When I wrote my first book and talked about eating fish and cheese, I found out really quickly that many raw foodists are militant when it comes to being vegan. And I am sorry, but I was not writing my book just for other raw foodists. Devoted raw foodists don't need to be told why raw food is so great or what the health benefits are, or how amazing they are going to feel, or what my results were. They know firsthand. I wrote my books first and foremost for newbies: people who had not yet found the benefits of raw or who may have hesitated to go raw because they were afraid of "failing." There is no failing.

Either you ate a meal raw or you didn't; and if you didn't, then you can eat the next meal raw. It is that simple.

it's easier than you think

This may sound like a bold statement, but I'll say it anyway: Going raw just may be the easiest thing you've ever done. It's not a diet plan like Weight Watchers; you don't have to count calories—in fact, I've never counted calories since I started eating raw. The benefits of adding more and more raw food to your meals will speak for themselves: I believe you will have more energy, your weight will be under control, and you might even heal yourself of a health condition or two.

But if you happen to eat something cooked one day, no big deal—pop a digestive enzyme and just get back on raw. When I cheat, it's something I plan for, and don't feel guilty about. Don't underestimate the value of a good attitude!

I accept that you may fear change; we all do. I will knock down those fears with some fun and daring. I challenge you to be healthy! I challenge you to give up your stomach acid, colds, and headaches for a life in which you may actually feel healthy.

the primer i've always wished i had

As the raw community continues to grow (and it is growing by leaps and bounds), I continue to learn, explore, collect, and come up with new recipes. In this book, I have included more than a hundred new favorite recipes. In fact, in addition to my easy, tasty new recipes, I have more than ever to share with you—a shopping list, a swapping list, tips, and extensive resources—that will make going raw that much easier. Although this is my third book, with all these added resources I consider it a primer—the primer I wish I had had when I started out! (Of course, the recipes are for everyone; newbies and seasoned pros alike will appreciate how easy to follow, creative, and satisfying they are.)

My aim is to give you the freedom to get creative in the kitchen while going raw at the pace that's best for you. After you've taken a look at my fantastic new recipes, you will get the "easy" part of the title, and you will be hard pressed not to go raw. Is this a challenge? You bet it is! And remember, not everyone likes everything! Raw food is like cooked food in that way.

how to use this book

Before you head into the kitchen and get out your chef's knife, I suggest you read through the first section of the book, Uncooked 101: What You Need to Know to Go Raw, to familiarize yourself with the basics. The section includes a chapter on how to tell what's really raw, a primer on raw equipment, and an A-to-Z shopping list.

The second section, the Methods, explains the techniques of soaking and sprouting, dehydrating, fermenting, and juicing.

The third section includes information on incorporating dairy and other animal products into the raw diet and how to shop for them. It explains how important fats are to your body and brain, dispelling the whole low-fat myth (in fact, I often eat half of my daily calories in fats alone!). In addition, this section covers all you need to know about choosing quality sweeteners, salt, and other staples.

I've also included a chapter called Turn It Raw (page 63). Most people tend to make the same things over and over again and shop for the same foods. But let me tell you, just about anything you make cooked, you can make raw. I'll teach you how. Turn It Raw shows you how to read a recipe and make it a little raw, half raw, or totally raw. Then, of course, there are the recipes. If you think raw means hours spent in the kitchen, think again. My recipes are not elaborate raw preparations—they are simple, delicious recipes highlighting fresh produce and other wholesome ingredients.

I've added a bonus chapter with a swapping list (page 234), as there is so much more raw out there than when I first started writing. More restaurants, yes, but also more prepared and packaged raw foods and online products. The swapping list takes traditional favorites such as chocolate, granola, and ice cream and helps you find their raw twin. Once you know what substitutes exist, your way of thinking will change, and you'll know what to reach for when you shop and when you prepare your food.

Finally, the online raw world has exploded in a parallel universe to the world of regular, old cooked prepared foods. I'll help you navigate online raw shopping with my extensive resources section (page 239). Try ordering some packaged foods so you can get an idea of what's available; you'll find it so much easier to stay raw when you have a little help, especially when you're out all day or on the road and don't have access to your raw-equipped kitchen.

going raw, going local

Since I started writing about raw, three words—"local," "seasonal," "organic"—have become a movement. Countless books have been written about eating in a more healthful and sustainable way. And it's easier than ever to eat good produce now, thanks to the growing number of farmers' markets, sprouting up throughout the country. But before we had farmers' markets, we had plain and simple supermarkets, and you won't lose points in my book if you shop at one. I salute you for eating your fruits and veggies, any way you can (as long as they are raw!).

In New York I tend to rely on Whole Foods and Fresh Direct, but you don't have to live in a big metropolitan area to go raw. My coauthor, Leda Scheintaub, can attest to that. She recently left the big city for the hills of Vermont, and with a little help from the Internet (see Sources, page 239), she has tested all of the recipes in this book with ingredients from her local natural foods store, supermarket, and farmers' market. And she picks up her milk (raw, of course) and eggs directly from her local dairy farmer and can go right to the farm for whatever produce is in season. She made her raw food searches a family outing. So can you!

in closing

I say this all the time, and I'll say it again: You don't have to be 100 percent raw. I know you are human, and no human being on earth can be 100 percent anything. Just because you can't give up your morning coffee yet doesn't mean you should give up on the whole thing. If you think you can do close to 100 percent, go for it, but don't become a martyr or a crusader. You'll just become annoying to your friends and family, and chances are you won't stick to it. Shoot for 75 to 95 percent raw—75 percent at first, and then aim upward toward that 95 percent—as this is when your body will see some serious changes for the better. Try it and see how wonderful you feel.

I'll leave you with a bit of insight: Let's face it, great food, whether we admit it or not, can be equal to or better than sex. Eating is a sensual experience that's all your own; you can watch TV while you do it, clean up whenever you want, with nobody else to please! So enjoy and eat up. This is gourmet dining at its best—and most delicious.

uncooked 101: what you need to know to go raw

Most people are confused by what *uncooked* means. Relax, I'm not asking you to give up cookies for cookie dough (by the way, the dough is *not* raw if you use sugar and processed flour!). I'm telling you to have your cake and eat it too—just eat it in the raw. Here are the basics—what you need to know and what you need to have—to get you started on the road to raw.

how to know what's really raw

Take a look at your food. How much of it do you really think is raw? Let's go over a few common culprits—foods that are often considered to be raw but aren't:

- **Salad:** This is where a lot of people get tripped up. What could be more raw than a salad? you ask. Well, the greens clearly are raw, but the croutons? And beans? Hard-boiled eggs? We'll help you figure out what's what.

- **Salad dressings:** Let's not forget about what you put on your salad. Whether you're having dressing at a restaurant or pouring it from a bottle, even if it's from the refrigerator or produce section of your supermarket, chances are it isn't raw. If the oil isn't cold-pressed (and it is a safe bet that it isn't, as it costs more), it's not raw. And that gourmet vinegar, unless it's raw apple cider vinegar, probably isn't raw either. That's why I have no shame and carry my own dressing with me (for more information, see the Salads & Salad Dressings chapter, page 121).

- **Hummus:** Say the label reads chickpeas, sesame seeds, olive oil, lemon, and salt. Sound good? Well, unless it's packaged with a label stating that it is raw hummus, those chickpeas are going to be cooked,

the sesame seeds may or may not be roasted (which means cooked), you can assume the olive oil is cooked (or it would say cold-pressed), and the salt most likely is table salt, which is highly processed. On the bright side, the lemon probably is raw. (Don't fret—see my all-raw hummus recipe on page 66.)

- **Sprouted bread:** In cases like this one, sometimes you really have to be a detective. Some brands that claim to be sprouted do this sneaky thing: The large writing on the front label says "SPROUTED." Now read the small print on the back—the first, second, and, if you're lucky, even the third ingredient may be sprouted. But after that, it usually has the same ingredients as any other loaf of bread. So you don't get all the benefits of sprouting, and you're paying twice the price of regular whole-wheat bread. We'll show you which breads are truly sprouted and how to make your own.

- **Chocolate:** Let's not even go into what is commercially done with chocolate! Chocolate melts at a relatively low temperature, so the chocolate itself usually isn't the culprit; it's what they add to the chocolate—often pasteurized milk, cooked sugar, and wax—that are the problems. Luckily, there are some great raw alternatives out there (see Sources, page 239).

- **Canned and frozen food:** Pretty much anything out of a can or jar is cooked, like pickles, chickpeas, and olives, for example. Even frozen vegetables are suspect—usually they are blanched (briefly cooked) before freezing. If you are unsure, go to the product's Web site or call up the company before committing to a purchase. It is just better to know than to think you are eating raw but not getting the results you were hoping to get, and wondering why.

Misconceptions abound on what is raw; here are a few common ones:

- **If it's cold, it's raw, isn't it?** No, raw is not the same thing as cold, as we saw in the deli hummus example above.

- **Isn't ice cream raw?** Sorry, no—the milk and cream are pasteurized. See Real Dairy and Eggs, page 48, to learn more.

- **How about yogurt?** Yogurt is cooked, too; even if it is made with unpasteurized milk, the milk is heated to make the yogurt.

- **And cheeses?** They are only raw if it says "made with raw milk" on the label. These you can buy in the store—you just need to know what to ask for.

Since I wrote my last book, the world has changed and so has our food. And, well, that is one of the reasons I am writing this book! I wanted to warn you that some products that were labeled "raw" are no longer raw, and you might not even know it. The label is exactly the same, sans the word "raw."

Case in point: agave nectar, the sweetener of choice for many raw foodists. Check the label—it's possible that the brand you bought last month has an identical label, tastes the same, costs the same. But it may not be the same—where is the word "raw"? Missing in action. The manufacturer might have changed its production methods (most likely to save money). You figured it out and looked online for another brand. Good job, Sherlock.

It doesn't stop with agave. As the raw foods industry continues to grow, shortcuts abound. Mass production has been introduced and so has radiation. Keep on your toes and check your labels periodically. If a label changes suddenly or you're not sure if something is raw, don't hesitate to call the manufacturer for a straight answer. I did just that with Bragg Liquid Aminos. Raw foodists use liquid aminos in place of soy sauce and in any number of dishes for flavor, but I no longer do. One day I noticed that the word "raw" wasn't on the label. A phone call to the company confirmed that, in fact, it was no longer raw. Now I use a new all-raw product called coconut aminos, made from the sap of the coconut tree (see Sources, page 239).

The lesson learned: Aside from fresh produce and raw grains, seeds, and nuts (minus the pasteurized almonds), it's pretty safe to assume that if the label doesn't say "raw," it isn't. Fear not— the shopping list on page 31 will help inform you on how to equip your raw kitchen with the staples that you'll use again and again.

warm it up— just don't kill it!

Even though raw foodists don't cook their food, not all raw food is served at a just-out-of-the-fridge temperature. Here are some tips on taking the chill off your raw food.

- **Warm it on the stovetop:** You don't have to serve your raw drinks and soups refrigerator cold unless you want to. Heat them until they feel just warm to the touch, or test them with an instant-read thermometer and make sure it doesn't go past the 110°F mark (here I say 110°F rather than 115°F because the temperature can continue to rise a little after you take your liquid off the stove).

- **Just don't boil it:** I know, you are used to boiling everything and then waiting for it to cool down to warm or room temperature before drinking it. Well, just skip the boiling step and go to the warm or room temperature step from the get-go. This will become a habit soon enough, and it will also save you time. This is good to know for making herbal teas, but not canned soups, which are already cooked.

- **Warm it up with oils:** Hot soups might give you the sweats and warm you up temporarily on a cold day, but that is a quick fix that fades just as fast. Adding raw oils to a raw soup, now that's hot! Raw oils help rebuild your body, and if you eat enough raw oils, your body will heat itself.

- **Take it out of the fridge:** Serve your foods at room temperature—take your pâtés, dips, and cheeses out of the refrigerator an hour or so before eating so their flavors will be at their fullest.

- **Dehydrate it:** If you're a raw foodist, you don't bake your food. But that doesn't mean you can't dehydrate it, as long as you keep the temperature at 115°F or under. See page 40 for more on dehydrating.

Look outside of the box—and your oven. Come on, don't be stubborn— there are endless ways of eating without cooking.

---

in other words . . .

COOKED
- baked
- blanched
- boiled
- broiled
- fried
- irradiated
- microwaved
- pasteurized
- refined
- roasted
- sautéed
- steamed
- toasted
- ultra-pasteurized

RAW*
- cold-pressed
- crude/*cru*
- dehydrated
- live/living
- (obviously) raw
- sprouted
- unpasteurized

* (but remember to check all the ingredients on your labels)

raw equipment: what you really need (and some fun gadgets)

I've got good news: Setting up your raw kitchen is as easy as one, two, three. Three appliances—a high-speed blender, a juicer, and a dehydrator—and your kitchen is ready to go raw. As you add more recipes to your repertoire, you may want to pick up some additional gadgets like a spiral slicer to make raw noodles or a mandoline to make vegetable chips. See what you like to make and you will figure out what you need.

Those top three appliances aren't cheap, but I promise you the payoff will be huge. You will make back your initial investment before you know it on the money you save on packaged food and takeout. And soon enough you will be churning out soups, pâtés, pastries, and more like a superstar chef.

High-Speed Blender: Your Kitchen's Workhorse

As you look through the recipes in the pages that follow, you will see that many of them call for a high-speed blender. If your morning smoothie is the toughest thing your blender is going to tackle, you may be fine with a standard kitchen model. Once you get more into raw, though, you're going to need a blender with some serious muscle.

I like the Vitamix blender; regular blenders generally range from 300 to 600 watts, but the Vitamix boasts 1,400 watts. It can juice a carrot, turn nuts into butter or milk, and blend a silky-smooth soup (and heat it up at the same time). The Vitamix is pricey (upward of $500), but it comes with a seven-year warranty and is built to last. I have had mine for ten years now and the motor runs as strong as the day I bought it.

When shopping for a blender, my advice is to check out the reviews and make sure it is powerful—at least 1,000 watts—and has a decent warranty. If you're mostly preparing food for one, there is another blender option for you that's reasonably priced: the Magic Bullet. It is petite, with a separate power base and blender cups—a small one for dips and such, and a tall one for smoothies, and extra "party mugs" to make smoothies to order when you're entertaining. It's smaller than a typical blender, so it's great for travel. But the best thing about the Magic Bullet is that it has a juicer attachment that allows you to make a fresh-pressed juice for one with virtually no cleanup.

> **tip**
> Check the Vitamix Web site for refurbished models.

Juicer: To Your Health

Juicing is one of the best things you can do for your body (see the Juicing section, page 45). Whole raw vegetables can be hard to digest. Juice those guys, and your stomach will thank you, especially when you first transition to raw. I used to get all my juices from a juice bar, but juices start to lose their "juice"—they oxidize and lose nutrition—within about twenty minutes of being exposed to air, so taking one to go for later wasn't an option.

Now I juice at home with a Jack LaLanne Power Juicer. It's powerful, and best of all, at around $100 it's one of the more affordable juicers on the market. The Jack LaLanne is a centrifugal juicer. The fruits and vegetables get shredded to a pulp, the pulp spins at a super-high speed, and centrifugal force presses the pulp against a strainer screen, so the juice pours into your glass. A big plus for the centrifugal juicer: It is quick and easy to use and clean up; my daily carrot juice takes four minutes to make, including cleanup.

Centrifugal juicers are your best and most affordable bet if you are doing a lot of fruit and carrot juicing, but they aren't built for large amounts of tough, fibrous leafy greens like kale or wheatgrass (they clog the basket). For that you will need a twin-gear press, such as a Green Star. This is the most expensive type of juicer, in the $500 range, but those twin gears work at slow speeds to extract large volumes of juice while keeping most of the nutrients intact. They also make nut butters, instant frozen desserts (pass a frozen banana through and you have banana ice cream), and fresh baby food (think of how much money that will save you).

Then there's the masticating juicer, which chomps down on your food and literally squeezes out the juice. The Champion, which has been around since 1954 and is in the $250 range, is one of the more popular brands. Though masticating juicers have just a single gear, they are very powerful; they can do much of what the twin-gear machines can do, with the exception of wheatgrass and large amounts of tough leafy greens.

Dehydrator: Your New "Oven"

Since oven temperatures don't go as low as 115°F, you will need a dehydrator to make raw cookies, crackers, main dishes, and more. To learn more about dehydrating, see the section on page 40.

There are a lot of food dehydrators to choose from, but the one that raw foodists go for is the Excalibur. It will cost you somewhere around $200 and it is fairly big, but it really is the best on the market. What makes it stand out is that it has removable trays—there is a five-tray and a nine-tray version—which gives you a lot of flexibility, including space for making several different recipes at once. If you want to make a casserole in a baking pan, just remove a couple of the trays and you will have all the clearance you need.

If your dehydrating needs are simple and limited to drying fruits and vegetables, a cheaper version might work for you (you can get one for $50), but make sure it has a reliable thermostat so you can keep your temperature at 115°F or lower. Some are limited to "high" and "low," and others don't have a thermostat at all.

ParaFlexx: Another word you can add to your culinary vocabulary. When you used to bake, you lined your pans with wax paper or parchment paper; now you will be lining your dehydrator with ParaFlexx sheets. These reusable sheets are made from nonstick material and keep liquid and spreadable foods from dripping through the dehydrator. Your dehydrator also comes with mesh screens, which are to be used for solid ingredients like fruits and vegetables. (ParaFlexx is a new name for what used to be called Teflex. It's the same thing.)

Food Processor:
A Handy Tool for Grating, Shredding, and Slicing

Your Vitamix, with its super powers of speed and strength, can do much of what a food processor can do. But a food processor can also slice, shred, and grate, and most models come with attachments for all of these operations. And for anything that is more solid than liquid, from pâtés to nut butters, a food processor can do the job quite well. Choose a food processor with at least 650 watts and a capacity based on your needs: A full-size food processor typically holds fourteen cups, a midsize holds seven to eleven cups, and a mini–food processor, which is an affordable, space-saving option if you are working with small amounts of food, has a three-cup capacity.

Coffee Grinder:
For the Little Jobs

The food processor isn't designed for small chopping and grinding jobs; that's where the coffee grinder comes in. Because it's so small (the food has more contact with the blade and less time flying around the machine) and strong, it can pulverize small amounts of nuts or spices into dust and chop tough chunks of raw hard cheeses like Parmigiano-Reggiano. A few tips: If there is a coffee drinker in the house, keep a separate grinder for raw ingredients or everything you grind will smell like coffee (and the coffee won't taste so great either). Take care when cleaning your grinder: Never immerse anything but the cover in water; and wipe the inside clean with a damp cloth followed by a dry towel. To thoroughly clean your coffee grinder, run a spoonful of flax seeds through it to pick up any remaining crumbs or spice residue.

If you have the Magic Bullet (see page 27), you'll be able to use its grinding attachment. So no need for a coffee grinder—unless, of course, you have not been able to give up your morning coffee . . .

Kitchen Thermometer:
For Those Who Like It Hot

If you crave the comfort of a hot bowl of soup or mug of milk, you can heat it on the stovetop until it feels warm to the touch—pretty simple. But if you don't quite trust your judgment or you want to get your food as hot as possible without killing it (you may be surprised at how hot 115°F is!), a $10 candy thermometer is an inexpensive and simple tool to use. Just clip it on the side of the pan; the thermometer will stay in the pan as your food comes up to temperature.

An instant-read thermometer can also be placed directly in the food to take a reading, but there is a downside: despite the name, it can take up to thirty seconds to give a reading, and by then the temperature may have risen too high. Before you know it, your food is cooked.

The most precise option, though a little more expensive, is a no-contact infrared thermometer. It is fun to use: Just aim and pull the trigger and you get a truly instant temperature reading without physically touching the food.

Spiral Slicer: For Pasta Lovers

The spiral slicer, also known as a spiralizer, is the tool for making raw noodles. This hand-cranked device was originally designed to make garnishes, but raw foodists have taken ownership of it: Run vegetables like zucchini, butternut squash, or sweet potatoes through it and you have instant pasta. A simple spiral slicer will cost you under $30. Most models have two settings:

one for angel-hair (thin) pasta and the other for wide noodles.

Mandoline:
Getting a Little Fancy

Not everyone needs a mandoline slicer, but if chips are your weakness, you might want to invest in one. Making your own chips in the dehydrator will save you money and keep you from snacking on fried—that is, cooked—chips. The mandoline will cut your food into even, paper-thin slices, and most mandolines also come equipped with interchangeable blades that make nifty waffle cuts, crinkle cuts, and julienne slices. Even a chef with the sharpest knife skills can't match the precision you get with a mandoline. You don't have to invest in an expensive stainless-steel French mandoline; save your money and opt for a cheaper plastic V slicer. Good brands include German-made Borner and Japanese-made Benriner, which you can get for under $50. Whichever model you choose, make sure it comes with a safety guard to keep your hands from making contact with the blade.

Yonanas: Just Plain Fun

As we were going to press, I discovered this gadget, which is a dedicated frozen fruit treat maker. Pass through bananas or other frozen fruits and you have an instant frozen dessert. It runs about $50 and is relatively small—a good option if you don't have a juicer or you don't want to lug it out every time you get the urge to make ice cream.

Vacuum Storage System (VacSy): Keeping Things Fresh

I love the concept of VacSy: It is a food storage system consisting of glass containers and a small, handheld vacuum pump that allows you to suck the air out, creating an oxygen-free environment that preserves your fruits, vegetables, and leftovers four to five times longer than regular glass or plastic containers. If you like to do a big shop and schedule your meals in advance, a VacSy can be very useful. The price tag is high, no getting around that, up to a few hundred dollars, but think of all the money you lose over the years tossing food that has passed its prime.

Sprouter: You Can Make Your Own

There are multiple options for sprouting—sprouting trays, sprouting jars, sprouting bags—all of them fairly inexpensive. I sprout my beans in a plain ol' jar or bowl and cover it with a new stocking so bugs can't get in. See page 36 for instructions on sprouting.

The Small Things: For an Efficient Kitchen

To keep things running smoothly, equip your kitchen with a nice assortment of knives (you will need a strong one for cracking coconuts), peelers, graters, spatulas, strainers, cutting boards, wet and dry measuring cups, and measuring spoons.

kitchen-ready: your a-to-z raw shopping list

Now that you've figured out what equipment your kitchen needs, let's put some food in it! This shopping list covers your basics: the foods you will find in a supermarket or natural foods store that you will be buying again and again. What it doesn't cover is hard-to-find specialty items and packaged foods; those products are on my Swapping List (page 234) and in Sources (pages 239).

What I'm Not Suggesting You Do

I'm not telling you to go out and buy everything on this list, and I'm not telling you to head to gourmet stores or natural foods stores every time you shop.

REAL-WORLD SHOPPING

The local, seasonal, organic movement is all the rage. That's great. But if that's more of an ideal than a reality for you, go ahead and shop at the supermarket, just like I do! True, you'll need a trip to your natural foods store to stock up on some essentials, but once you're set, the supermarket will serve you just fine for your fruits and veggies, fish, cold-pressed olive oil, and beans, nuts, seeds, and raisins from the bulk bin.

shopping list

DAIRY AND EGGS

- Raw milk (if your state allows it; see page 49)
- Raw-milk cheeses
- Fertilized organic eggs (farmers' markets)

NUTS, DRIED FRUITS, VEGETABLES, AND LEGUMES

- Brazil nuts
- Cashews
- Dried sea vegetables, such as nori, wakame, and dulse
- Macadamia nuts
- Nut and seed butters (raw), such as almond, cashew, and sesame tahini
- Pecans
- Pine nuts
- Pistachios
- Walnuts
- Chia seeds
- Flax seeds (light or dark)
- Hemp seeds
- Pumpkin seeds
- Sesame seeds
- Shredded dried coconut (not toasted)
- Sun-dried tomatoes
- Sunflower seeds
- Seeds for sprouting, such as alfalfa, broccoli, and radish
- Assorted dried fruit, such as apricots, figs, cherries, cranberries, and mangos
- Dates (preferably Medjool)
- Dried goji berries (unsweetened and unsulfured)
- Raisins
- Assorted dried beans
- Dried chickpeas
- Dried lentils

GRAINS

- Buckwheat
- Millet
- Oat groats
- Quinoa

OILS

- Cold-pressed extra-virgin olive oil
- Cold-pressed sesame oil
- Raw virgin coconut oil
- Udo's Choice Oil Blend (my choice for salads), flax oil, or hemp oil

FROZEN FOODS

- Ezekiel 4:9 and Genesis 1:29 breads, tortillas, buns, and English muffins (not raw, but sprouted—a bridge food)
- Manna bread (another bridge food—cooked on the outside but raw on the inside)
- Organic frozen fruit without syrup (for smoothies)

SWEETENERS

- Coconut nectar or coconut crystals
- Liquid or powdered stevia
- Rapadura
- Raw agave nectar (see page 53)
- Raw honey

SPICES, SEASONINGS, AND MISCELLANEOUS INGREDIENTS

- Green powder
- Nama shoyu (unpasteurized soy sauce) or coconut aminos

- Raw apple cider vinegar or coconut vinegar
- Raw cacao powder or carob powder
- Raw sauerkraut and pickles, such as Real Pickles or Grillo's Pickles
- Salt (preferably Himalayan salt or Celtic sea salt)
- Spices, such as cayenne, curry powder, cinnamon, nutmeg, and cumin
- Unpasteurized miso
- Vanilla extract and almond extract (alcohol-free)

CURED FISH AND MEAT

- Bresaola (cured beef)
- Gravlax (salt-cured fish; Spence and Co. is one of the only true raw gravlax brands on the market)
- Prosciutto (salt-cured and air-dried pork)

DRINKS

- Herbal teas
- Unpasteurized orange and other fresh juices (not from concentrate); I like the brand Just Pik't

SNACKS

- Raw bars, such as Go Raw, Organic Food, and Raw Revolution brands

FRESH PRODUCE

- Apples
- Asparagus
- Avocados
- Bananas
- Beets
- Bell peppers
- Berries, such as blueberries, strawberries, raspberries, and cranberries
- Bok choy
- Broccoli
- Cabbage
- Carrots
- Cauliflower
- Celery
- Cherries
- Chiles
- Coconuts (young)
- Cucumbers
- Endive
- Fennel
- Garlic
- Ginger

- Greens, such as chard, collards, kale, and spinach
- Herbs, such as cilantro, basil, rosemary, sage, and parsley
- Lemons and limes
- Lettuce
- Mangos
- Melons, such as cantaloupe, honeydew, and watermelon
- Onions
- Oranges
- Papayas
- Pineapple
- Radishes
- Scallions
- Sprouts
- Tomatoes
- Zucchini

NOTE: One staple is conspicuously missing from this list: almonds. As most of them are pasteurized (see page 59), you will have to buy them online from a source with a direct connection to the grower (see Sources, page 239) to be sure they are raw. Only raw almonds sprout.

What I *Am* Suggesting You Do

Health experts tell you to shop around the perimeter of the regular ol' supermarket, where you find the fresh foods, and shop carefully in the middle, where you find the packaged goods. I'll make it easier: Stick to one part of the perimeter, where you find the produce and fish (you can probably skip the dairy section, because the dairy products, with perhaps the exception of some cheeses, are pasteurized).

Set yourself up with a few basic items from your natural foods store—such as honey, nuts, seeds, and beans—so you have them on hand when a recipe calls for them. Then shop for your produce from the supermarket; it's quick and convenient, and I'll bet it will get you to eat your veggies!

eating the colors of the rainbow

Dr. Timothy Brantley, who taught me to eat raw, gave me this advice: Eat a wide variety of colors—not just greens—from a wide variety of foods. Yellow tomatoes, orange peppers, green avocados, red beets, purple cabbage, and so on. If you are eating eight avocados a day (or different recipes that all include avocados) and wondering why you aren't losing weight, it is because your body has stocked up on all those healthy fats from the avocado, and now you are imbalanced and top-heavy. My advice to you is not to give up avocados but to slow down and change up your colors—in a word, diversify!

the methods

Just because it's raw doesn't mean you can't get creative in the kitchen; you can make raw meals that feel cooked, have some crunch, and satisfy! If you're a gourmet, don't worry—you can go as fancy or elaborate as you like. If you're a dabbler, it can be as easy as blending. The methods may be new to you, but the main thing is to relax and have fun; I'll take you through it.

soaking and sprouting

Soaking, when called by its technical term, "germinating," tends to freak people out, but all "germinating" means is giving your nuts, beans, seeds, or grains a good soak, and sprouting is one step past germination. Soaking and sprouting are so easy because the legumes do all the work. Really! You just drop them in water, leave them there for a while, then drain and put them in a bowl to sprout.

There is no better example of what raw foodists refer to as "living" food than sprouts, as these little powerhouses of energy are still alive and growing when we eat them. And they are rich in fiber and very easy to digest to boot. You are probably familiar with alfalfa sprouts as the crowning touch on many a salad, and the mung bean sprouts that make their way into Chinese stir-fries. But you may not know that you can sprout just about any seed, grain, or bean: You can sprout chickpeas for raw hummus (page 66) or quinoa for a raw grain salad (page 174) to name a couple. When it comes to nuts, though, only almonds sprout.

Seeds, grains, beans, and nuts are filled with nutrition, but their life-giving nutrients are dormant, held back by enzyme inhibitors. They are like little Sleeping Beauties just waiting for you to wake them up. And all it takes to awaken them and release their many enzymes—along with vitamins, minerals, amino acids, and proteins—is to soak them and, if you wish, take the next step and sprout them for even more benefits. Soaking and sprouting also neutralize phytic acid—a substance found in seeds, grains, beans, and nuts—which keeps us from absorbing calcium, magnesium, iron, zinc, and other minerals. Many health-conscious people are familiar with phytic acid and its mineral-robbing properties, so they soak their grains and beans, awakening their food. But then they kill it by cooking it. Silly, huh? Don't make that mistake!

Each seed, grain, bean, and nut requires a specific amount of time to germinate (see chart, pages 38–39). To take it a step further, you can sprout them. The seeds, grains, or beans are drained and placed in a bowl or sprouter for an additional amount of time. They burst open and sprouts appear—a miracle of nature and a tasty, crunchy delight.

Germinating couldn't be easier:

1. Rinse the nuts, seeds, grains, or beans in a bowl and cover with filtered water in a ratio of about 3 parts water to 1 part beans. Cover with cheesecloth or a new stocking.

2. Refer to the chart on pages 38–39 for the soaking time, then rinse and drain. Your seeds, grains, beans,

tip

Freeze a stash of soaked nuts so you'll always have some on hand for your recipes.

or nuts are ready to use or to be sprouted.

To sprout, the method is always the same; only the time varies:

1. Follow the above instructions for soaking and place your soaked and drained almonds, seeds, grains, or beans in a bowl or wide-mouth jar. Cover the top with cheesecloth or a new stocking.

2. Leave your jar on the counter for the amount of time specified in the chart, rinsing the nuts, seeds, grains, or beans a couple of times a day with cool water to keep them hydrated and to keep mold from growing. Keep them well drained.

3. Rinse a final time and drain very well.

4. Place your sprouts in an airtight container and store them in the refrigerator for up to a week.

As I mentioned in the equipment section (see page 31), there are quite a few sprouters on the market, but I find a plain wide-mouth jar to be just as good, and if it's a clean recycled jar, it doesn't cost anything. And speaking of saving money, think of how much cheaper it is to sprout your own—the package of sprouts you buy at the supermarket for $3.99 would cost about 25 cents to make at home. And sprouts are pretty to look at, like a little countertop garden in a jar—now that's what I call eating locally!

TIPS FOR SUCCESSFUL SPROUTING

- **Start with the best quality raw almonds, seeds, grains, and beans:** Choose organic for the greatest health value.

- **Give your sprouts ample room to grow:** They will greatly expand as they sprout.

- **Don't let your sprouts become waterlogged:** Try putting your sprouting jar upside down at a 45-degree angle resting inside a bowl to allow for steady draining.

- **Give your sprouts lots of air:** If you find your sprouts getting soggy or turning bad before their time, try placing your sprouting nuts, seeds, grains, or beans in a strainer placed over a bowl for greater air circulation.

- **Keep the sprouting jar out of direct sunlight:** Too much sun can cause them to spoil.

- **Rinse more often in warm weather:** This prevents spoilage.

- **Dry your sprouts very well with paper towels before storing them in the refrigerator:** Try putting one paper towel on the bottom and another loosely on top of the sprouts in the storage jar to absorb any remaining moisture.

soaking & sprouting chart

FOOD	GERMINATION TIME	SPROUTING TIME
{ nuts }		
Almonds	8–12 hours	1–2 days
Brazil nuts	2 hours	n/a
Cashews	2–3 hours	n/a
Hazelnuts	2–4 hours	n/a
Macadamias	not necessary	n/a
Pecans	2–4 hours	n/a
Pine nuts	not necessary	n/a
Pistachios	not necessary	n/a
Walnuts	2–4 hours	n/a
{ seeds }		
Alfalfa	8–12 hours	2–5 days
Broccoli	8–12 hours	3–5 days
Clover	8–12 hours	4–5 days
Mustard	8–12 hours	4–6 days
Pumpkin	8 hours	1–2 days
Radish	8 hours	2–5 days
Red clover	8 hours	2–5 days
Sesame	8 hours	1–2 days
Sunflower	6 hours	2–3 days

FOOD	GERMINATION TIME	SPROUTING TIME
{ grains }		
Amaranth	8 hours	1–2 days
Barley	8–12 hours	2–3 days
Buckwheat	8–12 hours	2–3 days
Millet	30 minutes	1–2 days
Oat groats	8–12 hours	2 days
Quinoa	8 hours	1 day
Rye	8 hours	3 days
Spelt	8 hours	2 days
Wheatberries	8–12 hours	2–3 days
Wild rice	12 hours (see Note)	n/a
{ beans and other legumes }		
Adzuki beans	12 hours	3–5 days
Black beans	12 hours	3–4 days
Chickpeas	12 hours	2–4 days
Lentils	8 hours	2–3 days
Mung beans	8–12 hours	2–5 days
Pinto beans	12 hours	3–4 days

Note: Use only wild rice that is labeled "raw" (see Sources, page 239); raw wild rice only needs to be soaked before eating

slow cooking, aka dehydrating

If you are new to raw, the idea of dehydrating might seem a little intimidating. Well, just about anything can be intimidating if you let it, right? Some new ideas and words may not be part of your culinary vocabulary—yet. And dehydrating might seem like a totally new concept to you. But in reality the oven and the dehydrator are basically the same thing, but with an important difference: One cooks at a high temperature quickly, killing everything inside it; the other "cooks" at a low temperature slowly, maintaining life. In the dehydrator you can make your own crackers (for pennies), to-die-for cookies, nutrition-packed burgers, and home-made fruit leather. You can even dehydrate entire meals!

Dehydrating: it's really the simplest concept ever. It is the difference between a plum and a prune, a grape and a raisin—or a potato and a chip.

Yes, there are plenty of fabulous raw recipes you can make without a dehydrator, but why limit yourself? And yes, a dehydrator will take up a good chunk of real estate in your kitchen, but it will open up new worlds for you. Finally, while it's a pricey tool, this one-time expense will save you a lot of money in the not-too-long run. The Excalibur, which I recommend over any other brand (see page 28), costs around $200, but it will pay for itself many times over. That $4 bag of chips you just bought would cost you less than $1 in ingredients to make at home. You can make a bag of chips for the price of a potato, and a banana pancake for the cost of a banana. And you can easily double or triple the recipes you dehydrate so the food lasts you for weeks. Dehydrating requires a bit of advance planning, but little effort!

Here are some tips to optimize your dehydrating experience:

1. Always start with top-quality produce. Since the flavors will become concentrated (see number 6), you want to start out with the best.

2. Slice your foods uniformly. This will result in food that is evenly dehydrated and crisp; a mandoline can come in handy here.

3. Dip fruits in acidulated water (water with lemon juice) or citrus fruit juice. This prevents your fruits from browning.

4. Dehydrating concentrates your food. That is, it will shrink. For example, my "Popcorn" Cauliflower Crunchies recipe (page 223) calls for a whole head of cauliflower but yields just 2 cups of crunchies. That amount of deliciousness barely makes it off the ParaFlexx sheets before it is gone. So don't hesitate to double or triple

your recipes to fill up every one of your dehydrator's trays.

5. Water content affects dehydrating time. The higher the water content of a fruit or vegetable, the quicker the dehydrating time. And you can slice those fruits and vegetables thicker because they will shrink more. Strawberries, bananas, mushrooms, zucchini, and peas, for example, have a very high water content (as a guideline, think of how much a vegetable would shrink if you cooked it—back in the old days when you cooked your food).

6. Dehydrating concentrates flavors. Go light on the seasonings and salt before you put your food in the dehydrator, as the flavors will be more intense later.

7. Don't overthink your dehydrating times. There is a science behind dehydration, but it isn't an exact one. Adding ten minutes to an oven-baked recipe will dramatically change the outcome; in a dehydrator you can add an entire hour or two with only a subtle difference. It may take getting used to, so don't stress out if your flax crackers take twenty-five hours instead of twenty-four.

8. Account for the climate. High humidity can slow down the dehydration process; if you live in a damp climate or are dehydrating in the summer, you may need to tack some extra time onto your recipes.

9. Dehydrate your food evenly. Rotate your trays halfway through dehydrating and distribute your food evenly on the trays for the most consistent results.

10. Dehydrating makes your crackers and breads thinner. When you make crackers or breads in a dehydrator, their thickness will be reduced by half when they're done. So don't make them too thin, or they will be fragile and prone to breaking apart.

SLOOOW COOKING

I hear it all the time—preparing raw foods is time-consuming. Well, I guess that depends on how you look at it. But what if you look at your dehydrator as kind of a slow cooker, a really slow cooker? The slow cooker is so popular because you throw everything in a pot and go to work; then you come home and you have stew.

A dehydrator is the same concept: It might take 8 hours to dehydrate your pancakes, but you can whip up the batter in the evening and spread it over a dehydrator sheet, and in the morning your breakfast will be ready and waiting. Having a few people over tomorrow night? Slice some potatoes, toss with olive oil and salt, throw them on the tray, and the next day you can indulge your friends with homemade potato chips instead of opening a bag. How much easier—and cheaper—could it be?

11. Test for doneness. For fruit, cut a couple pieces in half; they should not be sticky, and you shouldn't be able to squeeze any moisture out of them. If you fold a piece in half, it shouldn't stick to itself. Vegetables should be dehydrated until they are brittle or crisp.

12. Test for doneness in more than one place. Foods tend to dehydrate faster at the edges of the trays than in the center, so test for doneness on more than one area of a tray.

13. Cool your food thoroughly after dehydrating: This ensures that there is no moisture remaining, so your food stays fresh. Store it in an airtight container to keep that moisture out.

14. Do not dehydrate chicken, meat, or fish. These foods do not suit our purposes here, with our maximum temperature of 115°F. It is not a temperature animal products like to hang out in—though bacteria love it. In the food business it is called the danger zone, and you don't want your meat to go there. When it comes to animal products, you've got to either kill it by thoroughly cooking it, or eat it raw (an exception is poultry, which I never recommend eating raw).

15. Keep your dehydrator clean. Wipe it with a damp washcloth every so often; check the bottom after each use and clean up any drips or crumbs so they don't accumulate.

the oldest form of cooking

Dehydrating isn't something raw foodists invented. In fact, the sun is our original dehydrator, and dehydrating is the oldest form of cooking and preserving known to humankind. It sustained many ancient cultures, from the Inca people to the Egyptians. In warm weather, food would be left out in the sun so the water would evaporate and the food would dry. The shelf life of the food would increase from a few days to the entire winter.

You, too, can experiment with sun drying during the summer months, when you have a surplus of tomatoes or other produce in your garden or if you go overboard shopping at the farmers' market or find a great sale at the supermarket. And if you live in the Southwest, you can sun dry most of the year. Just place your fruits or vegetables on a raised screen in a sunny spot, and cover them with another raised screen (to guard the food from critters while still providing ample ventilation). Let dry for several days, until leathery and pliable, bringing the food in at night to protect it from the morning dew. It's a bit more time-consuming than plugging in your electric dehydrator, but if you are a DIY or back-to-nature type, you may find it very satisfying.

16. Prepare your ParaFlexx sheets for the next round. Don't stack your sheets when they're wet; dry them thoroughly with a towel or place them in the dehydrator and run it at a high heat for about 30 minutes. Then your sheets are in place and ready to go for your next recipe.

17. Store your extra ParaFlexx sheets right at the bottom of the dehydrator. That will keep them out of your way; they won't be bothered by the heat when the machine is running.

18. Have fun. Get creative and do some experimenting. Don't worry—it won't burn!

At this point in my life, I wonder how I ever lived without my dehydrator. My coauthor, Leda Scheintaub, loves it so much that she has come up with a whole chapter just on dehydrator snacks, crackers, and breads (page 215). Snacking is fun, and I wouldn't dream of denying you your snacks just because you don't eat cooked food. Check out the recipes, and snack to your heart's desire.

fermenting

I like to think of fermented foods as alive, effervescent, immunity boosting, and health promoting. You can also call them pickled or cultured foods. But what these words do not tell you is that they are some of the healthiest foods you can eat and are a great addition to any raw foods lifestyle.

The ancient Greeks referred to fermentation as alchemy, and there is a bit of magic in the process. During fermentation, beneficial bacteria and enzymes break down a food, so by the time you begin eating it, the process of digestion has already begun. Raw vegetables can be difficult to digest, especially when you first go raw; adding fermented vegetables to your diet is one fantastic way to get the benefits of raw without the problem of bloat. You can also leave them sitting around the refrigerator so that they are available when you want them—they definitely don't go bad quickly! Fermentation also increases the flavor, nutrition, and enzyme levels of a food. Your body doesn't have to work as hard to absorb those nutrients, so you get more bang for your buck. See pages 108 to 111 for a couple of recipes.

So how do you get that bang for your buck? If you don't mind me getting

PICKLE JUICE DRESSING

Every jar of pickles comes with a bonus: pickle juice. Don't drain it when you've finished your last pickle—whisk a little into some cold-pressed olive oil and you've got an instant salty-sour dressing to toss your salads with. Or take a sip or two before a meal to jump-start your digestion.

a little scientific here, I will gladly explain: The principal by-product of fermentation is lactic acid, which promotes healthy intestinal flora and strengthens the immune system while preserving the food. (Okay, I am done being scientific—for now!)

From Eastern European sauerkraut to Korean kimchi, fermentation has played an important part in just about every traditional diet—except, unfortunately, the Standard American Diet, appropriately nicknamed SAD. We traded tradition for efficiency, as supermarket pickles and the like are often cured with vinegar and pasteurized to make them shelf stable, and they often contain sugar and preservatives to boot. All those friendly bacteria are killed off, so we lose the whole purpose of fermentation. At the end of the day, that pickle is no longer a nutritious food.

A vegetable that is fermented is wonderfully salty and sour and needs no adornment. And fermenting is a great way to keep produce long beyond the growing season. If you have a green thumb and like to grow your own veggies, you can eat out of your garden all winter long by fermenting your vegetables. When the supermarket has cucumbers on sale or your garden is overflowing with them, make Old World Cucumber Pickles (page 110); when there's an overabundance of carrots, try making some Ginger-Chile Pickled Carrots (page 108).

Just remember, there is a world of difference between a natural pickle and one you find on the supermarket shelf: Always look for the words "naturally fermented" and "raw" on the label to be sure you're getting the real thing.

But if you don't have the time to make your own fermented foods, you're in luck. When I first went raw, I couldn't find raw pickles or sauerkraut anywhere, but now there are a variety of brands to choose from and they can be ordered online, bought in supermarkets, or found in farmers' markets. Two of my favorite brands are Grillo's Pickles and Real Pickles (see Sources, page 239). And my simplest-ever recipe for borscht (page 148) involves little more than opening a jar of Real Pickles' raw pickled beets.

juicing

Fresh-pressed juices are incredibly easy to make and to consume; drinking them is one of the simplest and quickest ways of getting vitamins and minerals into your body. Juicing is also the fastest way to alkalize your system (see page 247 for more on pH) without putting stress on your body as the food breaks down and releases its nutrients. Your body doesn't have to make its own enzymes; it just takes the juice in and utilizes the enzymes (and those enzymes aid digestion), which makes juice a perfect part of any healing regimen. Just make sure your produce is top notch and you're good to go. I juice three times a day, but juicing once a day or even every other day will still do you a world of good.

As we get older, our enzymes get diluted and it becomes more and more difficult to digest vegetables, especially raw ones. Jack LaLanne was a shining example of what juicing can do for your health. The beloved father of American fitness lived ninety-six health-filled years, working out, swimming, and juicing every day.

What to Juice?

There is such a variety of possible juice combinations that you will never get bored; there are entire books on the subject. I love carrot juice. My boyfriend, Alexei, makes a fresh tomato juice, adds salt and pepper, and it's tomato soup in a glass. My friend Murray piles on the kale; he buys six pounds of it at a time and makes kale juice. Some people like to mix it up; at juice bars you'll often find combinations of five or six different vegetables and fruits on the menu.

A word of caution: Go easy on the fruits, which have a lot of sugar, and sweeter vegetables, like carrots and beets. Just because it's juice doesn't mean you can drink it with abandon. When you're juicing, you're essentially drinking condensed fruits and vegetables (four or five oranges in a glass of juice!) without the fiber to slow

---

for the best juices, start with the best produce

Don't skimp on quality when you're juicing. Pass on fruits or vegetables with bruises or that are on their way out. Juicing them won't disguise their poor quality. Pick fruits and vegetables that are ripe so you get a lot of juice out of them, but still crisp or firm so they pass through the juicer easily. And if possible, use organic produce—nothing irradiated, and no GMOs (see page 246). Juicing concentrates, and concentrated vitamins and minerals are what I want in my juice, not concentrated pesticides, thank you very much.

JUICE IT AND DRINK IT

Don't let your juice sit around after you make it. Drink it within twenty minutes, because after that it starts to oxidize, meaning it loses vitamins, minerals, and enzymes.

down the absorption of the sugar. And a big point of eating well is to keep your blood sugar balanced. To dilute sweet juice, add a neutral-tasting vegetable like cucumber or romaine lettuce to the juicer. Or dilute the juice with water—2 or 3 parts juice to 1 part water. Consume it slowly (though within twenty minutes) so the sugar doesn't hit you all at once.

You don't need me to tell you what juices to drink. You know what fruits and vegetables you like, and I'm confident that you can figure out your favorite combinations (and of course you'll never go wrong with a straight shot of a single type of juice). But in case you need a little jump-start, here are twenty wonderful combinations to inspire you to get juicing. You may be surprised by what kinds of produce you can juice!

1. Apple, parsley, and collards
2. Apple, pear, and cucumber
3. Blueberry, strawberry, and cucumber
4. Bok choy, spinach, and parsley
5. Cantaloupe, honeydew, and cucumber
6. Carrot, apple, and Swiss chard
7. Carrot, apple, cucumber, and ginger
8. Carrot, beet, and lettuce
9. Carrot, cabbage, and parsley
10. Carrot, parsnip, and spinach
11. Fennel, apple, and cucumber
12. Green apple, celery, and parsley
13. Kale, beet, and celery
14. Lettuce and red bell pepper
15. Mango, pineapple, cucumber, and lime
16. Papaya, pineapple, and cucumber
17. Pineapple, lemon, and lettuce
18. Tomato and celery
19. Tomato, cilantro, and garlic
20. Watermelon and mint

tip

Never look into the shoot you pass your vegetables through while the motor is running. If something like a seed or pit gets stuck, it can come shooting out with force and hurt you. Always turn off the machine before investigating.

really fresh juice doesn't come in a bottle

When I talk about juicing here, I always mean fresh-pressed juices. What you find in a bottle on the shelf at the market (surprise, surprise) is pasteurized (cooked) to keep it stable at room temperature. The bottles you find in the refrigerator section are also likely to be pasteurized (orange juice is often the lone exception), and even if they're not, they don't usually meet my criteria of fresh or nutritious (even if the labels say they're 100% juice). If you don't drink juice within twenty minutes after it's made, most of the valuable nutrients are oxidized anyway.

getting to know your food
(in all its raw glory)

I know, eating is something you've been doing all your life. So what can I tell you that you don't already know? Well, for one thing, over the past few decades our food has changed. And to be healthy you need to know your food. For me, as I explain throughout the book, the only way I know how to maintain my health is to eat raw.

real dairy and eggs

I love unpasteurized organic milk and I drink it whenever I can find it. The commercial dairy industry would have us believe that raw milk is unsafe, but I believe that any kind of organic milk (cow's, goat's, or sheep's) is as safe as the farm on which the animals were milked, be it a family farm or a factory farm. If you want to drink raw milk, know that it's controversial—and educate yourself!

Pasteurization—heating milk to a high temperature quickly—was introduced in the beginning of the twentieth century, for good reason. The world was urbanizing at a speedy pace, but production methods and dependable refrigeration were lagging, which led to outbreaks of food-borne illnesses and tuberculosis. But we have learned a thing or two about hygiene in the past century. Dairy farms have modernized: We now have stainless-steel tanks, milking machines, and refrigerated trucks, and raw milk is regularly tested for pathogens. Pasteurization increases the shelf life of milk, so that it can travel long distances before making it into your kitchen, and it often does. Why not keep it raw but keep it local? Just remember to buy from a farmer or retailer you trust, keep it cold, and don't keep it beyond the expiration date.

When it comes to good health for a raw foodist, nothing is more important than enzymes. Pasteurization obliterates pathogens, yes, but it also denatures milk proteins and destroys beneficial enzymes. No wonder digesting modern milk has its issues—it may have fewer digestive enzymes! Could pasteurization be why more and more people are becoming lactose intolerant? Many people who think they are lactose intolerant often are able to digest raw milk, so please consult your doctor if you are lactose intolerant and are thinking of trying raw milk.

Enzymes aren't the only thing that pasteurization affects. It also can break vitamin and mineral bonds, and destroys beneficial bacteria. I believe raw dairy is a health food, but you need to educate yourself about the type

DON'T MAKE PASTEURIZED MILK PART OF YOUR 5 TO 25 PERCENT NON-RAW ALLOTMENT

Remember how back in the Introduction I recommended shooting for between 75 and 95 percent raw? Because of all the issues with pasteurized milk—lack of digestive enzymes, possible added hormones, and lactose intolerance among them—I recommend that your 5 to 25 percent cooked food and drink *not* include pasteurized (cooked) milk. Worried about drinking raw? Skip the cow's milk and go for a nut milk (page 88).

of milk you'd like to drink. Raw dairy is referred to as "real dairy" by the Campaign for Real Milk, a group that provides information about the benefits of raw milk and promotes access to raw milk in every part of the country. The organization provides a state-by-state listing of farms that sell raw milk. Visit www.realmilk.com and click on to your state to find out the nearest farm. And while you're at the farm, for a real treat, see if it also offers raw heavy cream and raw butter; their richness and flavor are unlike anything you'll find in the supermarket.

Unless your local farm is down the road, you may want to stock up on raw milk and freeze it. Milk keeps for months in the freezer. It's a little gloppy (but still fresh) when it thaws, so save it for your smoothies and other blended drinks, rather than for your tea or for drinking straight. Freeze it in single servings for convenience.

An organization called the Farm-to-Consumer Legal Defense Fund is working on the legal aspects of consumer access to raw milk. Its Web site (www.farmtoconsumer.org) has a nifty color-coded map that provides a state-by-state review of raw-milk laws, as laws vary from state to state: In some states selling raw milk is illegal, in others you can buy it directly from the farm, and in still others you can buy it right in retail stores. (In some states raw milk is only legal to sell if it is marked as pet food!)

Raw-Milk Cheeses

French people are taught to look for the words "raw milk" on the label when they go to buy cheese, as they know that raw-milk cheeses are superior in quality and taste. Americans are taught to fear those same words, and by law cheeses sold in the United States must be pasteurized or aged for at least sixty days. The French insist that pasteurized milk cannot produce a cheese with character and complexity; cooked cheese just isn't French *fromage*. And they should know, as they have been eating raw-milk cheeses for centuries and developed a whole food culture around it.

As American raw foodists, the sixty-day aging requirement means we pass on fresh cheeses like soft goat cheese and we miss out on some fancy imported cheeses like Brie and Camembert, which you can readily find made from raw milk throughout Europe and even in Russia! But on the bright side, the law is clear—sixty days of aging and it can be sold, raw, in any state, right at the supermarket, unlike raw milk. What's more, a whole cottage industry of farmstead cheeses has sprouted up around the country, and American cheeses, like American wines, now compete on an international level.

To learn more about raw-milk cheeses or to find recommendations, go to the Raw Milk Cheesemakers' Association's Web site, www.rawmilkcheese.org. Or go to your supermarket or cheese shop and buy any cheese with the words "raw milk" on the label that looks good to you—simple enough! Since many people are actually looking for pasteurized, the labels are usually pretty easy to spot when it comes to raw-milk cheeses.

Kefir

Kefir is a cultured milk beverage, which means it's really good for you! Here I'll tell you why it's so good for you; on page 90 I will tell you how to make your own kefir using raw milk (or coconut water for vegans) and where to find the supplies you'll need.

Our kefir is like yogurt, only better, because it's not cooked and contains strains of beneficial bacteria that you won't find in yogurt—or any other food, for that matter. It looks like a thin, drinkable yogurt and it has a tart, refreshing flavor. And when you drink it, you just feel good (as a matter of fact, in Turkish *kefir* actually means "feel good").

A combination of bacteria and yeast grains are the starter; they form clusters that look like tiny cauliflowers. The grains can be used over and over again to make batch after batch of kefir, and over time they multiply so you can share them with others.

People need probiotics (beneficial bacteria), and the probiotics found in kefir are more numerous, nutritious, and therapeutic than those found in yogurt because they work to help predigest the foods you eat.

You will build up your immunity and clean out your digestive tract with kefir. While the bacteria in yogurt keep the digestive system clean and feed the friendly bacteria already there, the bacteria in kefir can actually colonize the intestinal tract, cleaning it out and helping to restore balance.

There's nothing more refreshing and nourishing than a glass of kefir or a smoothie made with it (page 76) first thing in the morning, and once you have your starter, making your own batch is a simple, inexpensive, and delicious way of doing good for your body.

Organic Eggs

In the food world little is more controversial than whether one should eat eggs raw. On the positive side, eggs

meat and fish: are they for you?

That's a complicated question, and the answer is a completely individual one, based on your beliefs, lifestyle, health, and genetics—I will leave that to you and your doctor to decide. But let me be clear: When it comes to eating your meat in the raw, I'm not telling you to eat it straight off the cow! You can "cook" your beef by marinating it (page 193); you can lightly sear your steak (page 70) so it is mostly raw; and you can pick up prosciutto (cured pork) or bresaola (cured beef) in the meat department. When it comes to fish, you can "cook" it in the form of ceviche (page 192) or cure it in the form of gravlax (page 154). You have many options. I generally recommend enjoying meat and fish in judicious amounts—as accents to your raw foods lifestyle rather than the main attraction.

A few tips: Shop for the best quality meat; "organic" and "grass-fed" are terms to look for on the label. And know your sources. If you can get to a farmers' market, you can connect with the farmer who raised the animals. Tell him or her that you are eating your meat raw and don't be afraid to ask questions. For fish, get to know the buyer at your fish store or supermarket and ask if the fish can be eaten raw (aka sashimi grade). Favor wild fish, as they have the highest levels of omega-3 fatty acids and a superior taste. Farmed fish are often crammed into close quarters and fed antibiotics, pesticides, and food with GMOs, and salmon may be fed artificial color pellets to make them bright pink. And remember, any canned fish is cooked.

are one of the best sources of protein around and one of the most nutritionally complete foods on earth. On the negative side, there is the possibility of salmonella, which is why the elderly, unwell, pregnant, or very young are cautioned to avoid raw eggs. And I would never recommend anyone eat a raw commercially mass-produced egg, as these facilities are where most of the outbreaks of salmonella seem to occur.

If you wish to take the chance and include raw eggs in your diet, the way I do it is with organic fertilized eggs, and by "fertilized," yes, I do mean after the cock has had his way with the chicken!

After fertilization the enzymes in the egg are released, which helps the chick to digest the concentrated yolk and release the nutrients, which makes them easy for us to digest and absorb, too. If these nutrients are good enough for the chick, they are good enough for me! And your eggs should be organic, because chickens that run free or eat no hormones or unhealthy feed create healthier eggs. Eggs that are both organic and fertilized are really your best bet. They make the freshest-tasting mayonnaise, and I like to crack one right into my salad (see page 133). If you're concerned about salmonella, you may choose to boil your eggs for just 2 to 3 minutes, so the whites and yolks are only partially cooked.

Unfortunately, organic fertilized eggs are usually found only in farmers' markets or right at the farm. I have learned that I have to fight for my organic fertilized eggs—they are usually sold out before eleven in the morning at my farmers' market!

sweeteners

We all need a little sweetness in our lives, so when you get the urge, choose raw sweeteners and try to pass on the refined sugars. With so many mouth-watering options to choose from—from tried and true honey, to supersweet stevia, to plain and simple dates—it won't be hard to do!

Rapadura

Rapadura is a fancy name for real brown sugar. It is produced by squeezing sugar cane. Then the juice is filtered and heated slightly (but within the parameters of raw), dried, and ground into sugar. It tastes like brown sugar, but the flavor is deeper, and it can be used as a substitute for commercial brown sugar in recipes.

Honey

Honey is nature's oldest sweetener; the only food that's sweeter is the date. As honey is sweeter than sugar, when you're converting your cooked recipes

RAW CANE SUGAR ISN'T RAW (AND NEITHER IS MOST BROWN SUGAR)

Raw cane sugar is a misnomer; it is more natural than regular white sugar, which is highly refined and bleached to remove its natural molasses. Raw cane sugar retains some of its nutrients and molasses, which gives it a darker color and distinct taste. But it's not raw—it is boiled and then dried as part of its processing. And most varieties of brown sugar (rapadura—see below left—is an exception) are just refined white sugar with a little molasses thrown in for color.

to raw, use a little less honey than you would sugar, and reduce the amount of liquid a bit.

What you may not know about this fabulous food is that it works as a natural preservative, so it adds to the shelf life of your recipes. Don't refrigerate honey; it should be kept at room temperature to prevent crystallization. If it does crystallize, set the honey jar in a bowl of very warm water and it will return to its liquid state. Crystallization is not harmful; in fact, it's a sure sign that your honey is raw.

When honey is pasteurized, it is perfectly clear and will stay that way virtually for eternity. But it has fewer nutrients and no enzymes, and therefore it is no longer a living food.

There are many different honeys to choose from, from mild and light clover and orange blossom to dark and full-bodied buckwheat. Lighter honeys have a more delicate, less assertive flavor and are the best choice for sweetening desserts; darker honeys have a stronger flavor and more depth. (Note that the FDA says honey of any kind isn't safe for babies under a year old.)

Agave Nectar

Agave nectar has become the go-to sweetener for raw foodists, particularly for vegans who do not partake of honey. It comes from a Mexican cactus, the same one that tequila comes from—but that doesn't mean tequila is part of the raw foods diet!

Read your labels carefully to make sure the brand you choose is raw. As I mentioned on page 25, some brands of agave that used to be raw no longer are. You may have to go online to find raw agave—but if you order in bulk, you can get some good deals (see Sources, page 239).

Your choices are light agave or dark (aka blue) agave. As with honey, light agave is also lighter in taste; it doesn't assert its flavor, so it works well in recipes where you want other flavors to shine. Dark agave, on the other hand, has a deeper flavor similar to molasses and can mask other more subtle flavors.

Like honey, agave is sweeter than sugar, so when you're going from cooked to raw, use a little less agave than you would sugar alone and reduce the amount of liquid a bit.

Dates

Dates originally hail from the Middle East, where they have been an important part of the region's cuisine for thousands of years. They can be eaten as a simple treat on their own or in place of other sweeteners.

In my recipes I recommend Medjool dates, known as the "king of dates," as they are the softest, sweetest, biggest, and juiciest dates—perfect for your raw food recipes. Other types of dates, such as Deglet Noor, are smaller, so if you use them, you may need to increase the number.

Stevia

Stevia, a noncaloric sweetener from the leaves of the stevia plant, has been used for centuries in South America and is very popular in Japan as an alternative to artificial sweeteners. It has a negligible effect on blood sugar. I find it tastes just like Sweet 'N Low, so if you are looking for a natural replacement for that neurotoxic sweetener, stevia is for you!

Up until 2008, stevia could only be marketed as a dietary supplement, but now it is also sold as a sweetener, and you will find it in natural foods stores and in some supermarkets in liquid or powder form (in convenient little packets similar to sugar packets). Choose the green or brown powder, as they are less processed than the white. Stevia is about two hundred times sweeter than sugar, so a little bit goes a long way—a drop or two in a cup of tea or your cereal is all you need.

Some find stevia has a bitter and licoricelike aftertaste not to their liking, though you can offset that aftertaste with citrus or tart flavors (see page 94 for recipes for drinks made with stevia).

Coconut Nectar and Coconut Crystals

Coconut as a sweetener? Yes! These products come from coconut but don't taste like coconut because they are made from the sap of the tree rather than from coconut meat. The sap is evaporated at a low temperature, and the resulting nectar is naturally sweet and very low on the glycemic index—lower even than agave. Coconut nectar is a rich, thick syrup, a bit like molasses in taste and mouthfeel. Coconut crystals are similar to brown sugar in taste and looks. Both sweeteners are wonderful sprinkled on cereal, pancakes, and the like or stirred into your tea. Coconut nectar and coconut crystals can be found in some natural food stores and online (see Sources, page 239). They are on the expensive side, so if you're on a budget, you may want to go for honey or agave.

Yacón Syrup

Yacón syrup, brown in color, thick in texture, and with a deep flavor similar to blackstrap molasses, comes from a root plant found in the Andes. It is low in calories and sugar, making it a smart pick for those of us watching our sugar intake. Our bodies cannot process the substance that gives it its sweet taste, so it passes through, leaving our bodies sugar free! And as an added bonus, yacón syrup contains healthy bacteria to support our digestive and immune systems. Yacón syrup can be found in some natural foods stores and online (see Sources, page 239).

seasonings

How you season your food can make or break a recipe. For example, salt doesn't just make your food salty—it also brings out the natural flavors in the food, and a dash of vinegar mellows the heat of a spicy dish. Use raw seasonings liberally to stir up memories of Italy, India, Mexico, or other countries of your choosing.

Salt

You can't survive without salt, but the type of salt you choose makes all the difference. Pass on the table salt— whether it's kosher or iodized, it is highly refined and heated to incredibly high temperatures, 1,000°F and up. Now that sure isn't raw! Trace minerals are stripped and anticaking agents containing aluminum are added to prevent the salt from absorbing the moisture in the air (yuck!). The aluminum leaves a bitter taste, so often sugar is added. And while it may be nice to keep the moisture away from your salt to keep it flowing, in our bodies the anticaking agents cause a similar effect. The salt doesn't dissolve in the fluids in our bodies, so it builds up and leaves deposits, which some health experts believe can lead to high blood pressure and heart disease. So stay away from refined salt to keep your blood pressure in check.

Sea salt is a whole different story. It is unrefined salt that is made by simply evaporating saltwater in the sun. What to look for on the label: a one-word ingredient list—salt, and nothing more—and the word "unrefined" on the label. Sea salt supports all our bodily functions, without the added chemicals found in table salt. And once you try it, you won't want to go back to refined salt: Sea salt is full of flavor with a slightly sweet aftertaste; refined salt has a sharp, chemical taste. While refined salt, much like refined sugar, is pure white, sea salt varies in color, from off-white or gray to pink or red.

Celtic sea salt, gathered from pristine waters, is gray in color and one of my favorites. But the crème de la crème of salts is Himalayan salt, from the remote Himalayan mountains. It often has a lovely pink color and it's the purest salt on earth. Both are available from natural foods stores and online (see Sources, page 239). They are a little pricier than other sea salts, so go for whatever sea salt fits your budget, as long as it is pure and unrefined.

Vinegar

As you read through the recipes in the pages that follow, you'll notice that I call for apple cider vinegar, coconut vinegar, and umeboshi plum vinegar, but not balsamic or wine vinegar; these last two generally aren't raw.

Apple cider vinegar, when it's raw (or unpasteurized) and unfiltered, will have a cloudy sediment at the bottom of the bottle. This is a good thing; it means it's the real deal. The sediment is part of the "mother" that created the vinegar and contains good bacteria and enzymes. Apple cider vinegar has a tart, crisp flavor and should taste like the apples it was made from. It is known to be detoxifying and good for your digestion. Use it in your salad dressings as you would balsamic or wine vinegar.

Coconut vinegar is another great option; like coconut nectar and coconut crystals (see page 54), it is made from the sap of the coconut tree. It is a little lighter than apple cider vinegar, with many similar healing properties. It has an acidic taste similar to rice vinegar and can be used as you would any other vinegar.

Umeboshi plum vinegar comes from a naturally pickled Japanese plum. It has a sour, tart, and fruity flavor. Although it's not considered a true vinegar because it contains salt, we use it as such for dressings (see my Easiest Umeboshi Vinaigrette, page 124).

Nama Shoyu

This is the raw version of soy sauce. Currently Ohsawa is the only brand offering raw nama shoyu in the United States. It is a fermented food, so it is full of enzymes and natural bacteria. Note that nama shoyu contains a small amount of wheat. If you are avoiding gluten, you might want to use wheat-free tamari. It's cooked (make it part of your 5 to 25 percent cooked!), but then it is fermented, so it is full of beneficial bacteria.

As I mentioned earlier, Bragg Liquid Aminos have been widely used in the raw community, but now they are no longer raw, and the label has changed. A call to the company confirmed that it is not a raw food. A newer all-raw option is coconut aminos, made from the sap of the coconut tree, which you'll find in natural foods stores and online.

WHEN IT'S SUGAR YOU'RE CRAVING, REACH FOR THE CIDER VINEGAR

When you're really jonesing for something sweet, before you grab for a candy bar, try this trick: Mix a teaspoon or two of raw apple cider vinegar in a cup of water, drink up, and wait a few minutes for the cider vinegar to cut through the craving. And if you add a teaspoon of raw honey, you have a traditional Vermont kitchen tonic for aches and pains or for a boost of energy when you need it.

Fish Sauce

Fish sauce is to much of Southeast Asia what soy sauce is to China and Japan, and it dates all the way back to Roman times. Fish—generally anchovies or sardines—are mixed with salt and water and left to ferment. The fermented juice that's left at the end of the process is the fish sauce.

Don't be intimidated by its rather stinky aroma: When you mix it with other ingredients, particularly lime (see my Thai-Style Mango Salad, page 159), it does a bit of magic and makes your food taste so much better, which is why it is ubiquitous in Thai and Vietnamese cooking. And since it is fermented rather than heated, that makes it a raw food! You can find fish sauce in Asian groceries and in some supermarkets in the international foods section.

Miso

This fermented bean paste is familiar to most of us as the base for soup served in Japanese restaurants. Most supermarket miso paste is pasteurized, but I find unpasteurized miso, which is a living food, with all the beneficial digestive enzymes that go along with living foods, right in my natural foods store. Add it to soups, dips, marinades, and dressings for a salty, earthy flavor kick. If your natural foods store doesn't carry unpasteurized miso, order it online (see Sources, page 239).

Sea Vegetables

Even if you think you don't like seaweed, you've probably eaten or used it—it's found in unexpected places like ice creams, salad dressings, even toothpaste and skin-care products. Seaweed might take a little getting used to for some people, but it is a nutritional powerhouse: Ounce for ounce, seaweed is higher in vitamins and minerals than any other type of food. So get to know seaweed, as a nori wrap for your tuna rolls (page 190), as wakame in a cucumber salad (page 138), or as dulse, a smoky-flavored sea vegetable, in a kale and avocado salad (page 137). Or sprinkle seaweed flakes over your food.

> **tip**
> To minimize the fishy flavor, soak your seaweed (and discard the soaking water) before eating it, or season it with lemon, lime, or raw vinegar.

Nutritional Yeast

Nutritional yeast is a nutrient-packed superfood that is high in vitamin B_{12}. It is also a complete protein. That's two important reasons for you—especially if you are a vegetarian or vegan—to sprinkle it on soups, salads, or snacks or add it to any number of dishes. Another reason is taste: Its nutty, cheesy, salty flavor enhances any savory food it's added to.

Choose a primary grown nutritional yeast, as this type of yeast is grown on mineral-rich molasses—the yeast takes in the minerals from the molasses and passes them on to you. My favorite brand is Quantum Nutritional Flakes (see Sources, page 239). You don't want brewer's yeast, which is a by-product of the beer-brewing industry and does not have the nutritional profile of primary grown nutritional yeast.

oils

....

When you shop for oils reading labels is key: For olive oil or sesame oil, look for the words "cold pressed" on the label; anything else is not raw. For coconut oil (also known as coconut butter), look for the words "raw," "expeller pressed," or "virgin" on the label. Coconut oil is solid when it's cold and liquid when at room temperature.

When it comes to getting in my essential fatty acids, Udo's Choice Oil Blend from Udo Erasmus is what I reach for. It contains all three fatty acids: omega-3, omega-6, and omega-9 (the "good" fats that are necessary for all bodily functions) and is a great pick for salad dressings or drizzling over any dish. You'll find it in the refrigerated section of your natural foods store, often in the supplement section. I recommend it because it is the oil version of eating a "wide variety." If you can't find it, look for another quality essential fatty acid oil blend.

As you can imagine, Udo Erasmus, author of *Fats That Heal, Fats That Kill*, knows a thing or two about oils, so I asked him why oils are so important for us. According to Udo, what a lot of people don't realize is that more health problems come from bad oils, and more health benefits come from good oils than from any other source. In fact, oils are vital to our health. People who are on very low-fat diets start noticing negative effects on their bodies, with symptoms such as dry skin and plummeting energy levels. If you don't get enough oils, over time the entire body begins to deteriorate.

And contrary to popular belief, Udo explained, oils don't make us fat. Of the essential nutrients that we need from foods, oils are the most crucial, and one of the most neglected. For example, about 95 percent of people are getting less omega-3 fatty acids than they need. This is because there are few good sources of omega-3s in the foods we normally eat, and on top of that omega-3s are extremely sensitive to damage by light, oxygen, and heat. The oils that we buy from the supermarket have been processed in a way that gives them a long shelf life. To do that, the oil manufacturers treat oils with harsh chemicals, then bleach them, and finally heat them to frying temperature to clean up the mess made by the chemicals and bleach. The resulting oils are not only odorless and tasteless; their molecules are damaged as well. This interferes with our health by changing how our genes function. A good rule to remember is that oils treat us like we treat them. If we treat them with care, they take care of us. If we damage them, they damage us. If we fry oils, they fry our health. On the other hand, if we favor raw foods, we'll automatically lean more toward healthful oils.

Udo is happy to report that after almost three decades of studying oils, numerous research studies have confirmed what he initially suspected: When we increase the amount of good oils in our diet, especially omega-3s, we can avoid or treat virtually every major degenerative condition of our time. Using an oil that provides enough omega-3s helps the body make powerful anti-inflammatory molecules and antioxidants, and omega-3 molecules have been shown to decrease the symptoms of autoimmune diseases.

Good oils can enhance mood and reduce stress levels, lift depression, ease the symptoms of major mental disorders, balance hormones, and help with learning problems. Supplementing with good oils has been shown to help performance in athletes and help with weight management. Good oils improve the absorption of nutrients and digestion, reduce carbohydrate cravings, and enhance the flavor of the foods they are used with. In addition, they improve the health of the skin, hair, and nails. And, finally, oils will do wonders for you in the bedroom—Udo says that supplementing with good raw oils supports the reproductive system and boosts libido. See, I told you that raw was sexy!

other staples

Bread

Don't pass that bread! If you're transitioning to raw or care to include a little bread as your cooked percentage (remember, I'm only asking you to go 75 to 95 percent raw), I've got two great ready-made options. (For you purists, skip on over to the raw bread recipes on pages 220 to 222).

Ezekiel bread can be found in the frozen foods section of your natural foods store. It isn't raw, but it's flourless and sprouted, so it is more easily digestible than regular bread and it's filled with vitamins and minerals and fiber.

Manna bread is cooked on the outside but raw on the inside and sprouted; it also is found in the frozen foods section. I love this as my lazy man's dessert: I buy the raisin-cinnamon bread, cut a slice, drizzle on a little honey, and grab my fork.

Nuts and Seeds

Good news: Many of the nuts and seeds you'll find in the bulk section of your supermarket or natural foods store are raw (as long as they aren't labeled "roasted" or "roasted and salted"). The unfortunate exception is almonds. In 2007 the FDA mandated that all almonds be pasteurized because of some salmonella outbreaks. Yet—here's the kicker—pasteurized almonds can still be labeled "raw." Manufacturers can do this when the almonds are flash-pasteurized (subjected to high temperatures for a short time). To raw foodists, if you flash-pasteurize, you still kill the enzymes, and the food won't sprout. Therefore flash-pasteurized foods are not considered raw. You can avoid the issue by buying almonds direct from the buyer (see Sources, page 239). Beware of imported raw almonds, as foods are regularly irradiated, the equivalent of nuking them, as they enter the United States.

To ensure your nuts are raw and make them more digestible, I recommend soaking, or germinating, them (see page 36). If they do not germinate (grow big and fat) or sprout (spring a little tail), they are not raw.

Flax and chia seeds play an important part in raw recipes for two reasons. Both are full of fiber, protein, vitamins, minerals, and omega-3 fatty acids. Flax seeds have amazing binding powers. When they are soaked, they become the base for the easiest crackers ever (see pages 216 and 217 for recipes). Chia seeds swell up to ten times their volume when soaked in water, making them the perfect hydrating food for athletes. They also thicken into a satisfying breakfast porridge (page 79). Or make a chia gel using 1 part chia to 9 parts liquid. Mix well, and allow 10 minutes for the seeds to fully hydrate. Use a little in salad dressings, smoothies, and the like to add some body. No wonder they are listed as one of nature's amazing superfoods.

Dried Fruit

Buy dried fruits that are labeled "raw"; others may have been dried at high temperatures. Make sure they are not treated with sulfur or sweetened with sugar. (See page 40 for drying your own.) Eat them as a sweet snack, in trail mix, or as a sweetener in desserts. Goji berries have become a popular fruit choice in recent years. In its dried form this little fruit is ruby red and the shape of a skinny raisin, and it is considered a superfood because of its amazingly high antioxidant content. Use them as you would raisins. You can find goji berries in some supermarkets, most natural foods stores, and online.

Coconut

In the raw food diet, coconuts seem to be a staple! They are used in just about every type of food—soup, noodles, creamy toppings, mousses, ice cream, and sour cream, to name a few. The coconuts I use are young coconuts, also known as Thai coconuts. They are soft and off-white in color with a pointed top—not to be confused with mature coconuts, the ones with the dark brown, hairy exterior and hard shell.

Young coconuts are the nutritionally superior coconut, and as they gain in popularity, more and more natural foods stores are carrying them. If yours doesn't, ask the produce department if they will order them for you. Or, if there is an Asian market nearby, you may find young coconuts there. The coconut meat and water freeze well, so one option is to buy them in bulk and get cracking (freeze the meat and water separately). Choose your young coconuts carefully: Avoid those with spots of mold; chances are they will be rotten inside. The water should be slightly cloudy, but still transparent; if it is pink, it is spoiled and should be thrown out.

Young coconuts are an important ingredient for raw foodists, for many reasons. Coconut water is filled with electrolytes and is high in potassium and other minerals (but avoid the coconut water you find on the shelf, as it's pasteurized). And young coconuts are full of healthy fats, including lauric acid, which works to speed up the metabolism and maybe even help you to lose weight! They also have antibacterial properties. But best of all, the coconut meat is utterly delicious and creamy, making it perfect for shakes, ice cream, soups, and coconut "noodles" (see the recipe on page 145).

{ how to open a young coconut }

Don't be daunted—it's easier than it looks, and with a little practice, it will feel completely natural.

Here's how to do it:

1. Stand the coconut on a steady, flat work surface.

2. Hold the side of the coconut with one hand, and using a heavy knife or cleaver, make a horizontal cut on the opposite side of the coconut about 1 inch below the tip, with the blade at a 45-degree angle (watch your fingers!).

3. Give the coconut a quarter turn and make another cut in the same manner, connecting the second cut with the first.

4. Give the coconut two more quarter turns, cutting each time, until you have cut a little square off the tip. Using the bottom of your knife's blade, pry the "cap" open.

5. Drink the water (pour it into a glass or pop a straw into the hole), or drain it and save it for a recipe.

6. Turn the coconut on its side and split it open with your knife: Hold the knife at a 45-degree angle so the bottom part of the knife's blade is making the cut. Give it a good whack so the knife gets stuck in the coconut; then whack the coconut on its side (with the knife still in it) until it splits in half. Spoon out the coconut meat.

turn it raw

I know it's hard to go cold turkey on anything. Raw food is no exception. Don't fear and don't fret. Let's try to get there slowly, but with the goal of adding more and more raw until you hit your healthy raw point. With some handy tips and the Turn It Raw recipes that follow, I will show you how to move more in the raw direction, and we'll have a blast while we're at it.

tomato salsa

If you're new to raw, let's start with something easy—tomatoes. There's nothing more flavorful than a just-picked raw tomato, and nothing better to make salsa with. Now, why would anyone want to cook that tomato? The answer: Because it's economical for manufacturers—jarred tomato salsa is cooked so it can be kept on the shelf for a long time. Luckily, making your own raw salsa only takes a few minutes. Here's how you go from cooked to raw, one step at a time.

cooked tomato salsa

Buy a jar of tomato salsa from the supermarket and open the lid!

partially raw tomato salsa

OPTION 1: Make your salsa with canned tomatoes, but use cold-pressed olive oil, lime juice instead of vinegar, sea salt, and raw onions and chiles to take a few steps in the raw direction.

OPTION 2: Make your salsa with regular olive oil (or omit the oil completely; it's not a must) and table salt, but use fresh tomatoes rather than canned.

4 medium plum tomatoes, seeded and chopped

½ small red onion, finely chopped

3 tablespoons fresh lime juice, or to taste

2 tablespoons cold-pressed extra-virgin olive oil

1 jalapeño chile, minced (seeded, if you like)

¼ teaspoon sea salt, or to taste

½ cup chopped fresh cilantro

totally raw tomato salsa

{ **MAKES ABOUT 1½ CUPS** }

Here's your complete salsa with a raw makeover. It is best the day it's made but will keep for a couple of days in the refrigerator.

In a medium bowl, combine all the ingredients except the cilantro and stir to blend. Taste and add more lime juice or salt if needed. Stir in the cilantro.

from cooked to raw

Once you get the hang of making adjustments, go through the pages of your favorite cookbooks, choose a few recipes, and use the principles below to start turning them partially raw or totally raw.

Let's begin with ingredients. Changing some of your ingredients from cooked versions to raw is an excellent place to start, as many ingredients are very similar and you'll barely taste the difference when you switch over.

COOKED INGREDIENT	TURN IT RAW INGREDIENT
Balsamic or wine vinegar	Raw apple cider vinegar or coconut vinegar (see page 56)
Bottled juice	Juice fresh from your juicer
Bread	Ezekiel bread or Manna bread (see page 59) for partially raw; for 100% raw breads, see the recipes on pages 220 to 222 or order from the Sources sction (page 239)
Extra-virgin olive oil	Cold-pressed extra-virgin olive oil (see page 58)
Miso soup packets	Unpasteurized miso paste (see page 57)
Pasteurized milk	Raw milk or Basic Nut or Seed Milk (see page 88)
Soy sauce	Nama shoyu (see page 56)
Table salt	Sea salt or Himalayan salt (see page 55)
Table sugar	Rapadura, raw honey, raw agave nectar, or coconut nectar (see page 52)
Yogurt	Basic Kefir (page 90)

hummus

When I first discovered that it was possible to make a raw version of hummus, my snacking life became so much easier. So much less guilty.

The hummus you find in little plastic tubs in the supermarket is made from cooked chickpeas unless it is specifically labeled raw. In addition to chickpeas, hummus is made with tahini, aka sesame paste, and more often than not those sesame seeds are roasted. Finally, a lot of oil goes into your hummus to make it smooth and creamy, and as you might have guessed by now, usually that oil is cooked.

Here's how to turn your hummus raw, step by step.

cooked hummus

Open a can of chickpeas, put them in a food processor, add regular tahini, cooked oil, table salt, and blend. Or just buy it in the store!

partially raw hummus

OPTION 1: Use canned chickpeas, but choose a raw tahini from the natural foods store, make your oil cold-pressed, and season with sea salt.

OPTION 2: Use sprouted raw chickpeas (see page 39) and regular tahini (or vice versa), and cooked oil.

totally raw hummus

{ **SERVES 4 TO 6** }

3 cups sprouted chickpeas (see page 39)

¾ cup cold-pressed extra-virgin olive oil

½ cup raw sesame tahini

3 tablespoons fresh lemon juice, or to taste

1 garlic clove, chopped

½ teaspoon sea salt, or to taste

2 tablespoons chopped fresh parsley or other fresh herb

Hummus without heating! And if you don't like chickpeas, or you want to change things around once in a while, use macadamia nuts or cashews instead of chickpeas. FYI: You'll need a high-speed blender to turn those tough uncooked chickpeas into raw hummus; otherwise you risk blowing out your motor!

In a high-speed blender, combine all the ingredients except the parsley and blend until smooth, scraping down the sides to move the ingredients around. Add water if needed to thin it out. Taste and add more lemon juice and/or salt if needed. Transfer the hummus to a bowl and stir in the parsley.

gazpacho

Good news: Gazpacho is a really easy cold soup to turn raw. The following is a typical ingredients list for a partially raw gazpacho. **Question:** Can you guess which ingredients might be cooked?*

partially raw gazpacho

Fresh tomatoes

Cucumber

Red onion

Red bell pepper

Garlic

Red wine vinegar

Fresh lime juice

Olive oil (not cold-pressed)

Fresh cilantro

Bottled tomato juice

Table salt

Now let's turn those ingredients around to turn our gazpacho completely raw.

2 large tomatoes, seeded and finely chopped

1 small cucumber, peeled, seeded, and finely chopped

½ medium red onion, finely chopped

1 small red bell pepper, cored, seeded, and finely chopped

1 garlic clove, pressed through a garlic press

1 tablespoon raw apple cider vinegar, or to taste

1 tablespoon fresh lime juice, or to taste

1 tablespoon cold-pressed extra-virgin olive oil

Sea salt

1½ cups freshly pressed tomato juice

½ cup chopped fresh cilantro

totally raw gazpacho

{ SERVES 4 }

In a large bowl, combine the tomatoes, cucumber, onion, bell pepper, garlic, vinegar, lime juice, oil, and salt to taste.

Transfer half of the vegetable mixture to a food processor or blender, add the tomato juice, and pulse to a chunky puree.

Return the puree to the bowl and stir it into the vegetables. Taste and adjust the seasonings, adding more vinegar, lime juice, or salt if needed.

Cover and refrigerate for at least 1 hour, until cold. Stir in the cilantro before serving.

*Answer: The cooked ingredients are red wine vinegar, olive oil, bottled tomato juice, and table salt.

pasta with tomato sauce

Everyone loves pasta, so it can be a challenge to give up the cooked stuff. But it doesn't have to be all or nothing—follow these tips so you can enjoy your pasta in any stage between cooked and raw.

cooked pasta with tomato sauce

Boil wheat spaghetti noodles and toss them with jarred or canned tomato sauce.

partially raw pasta with tomato sauce

OPTION 1: Cook your wheat pasta and tomato sauce, but add the olive oil (make sure it's cold-pressed) and salt (make it sea salt) last, so they remain raw. A little adjustment—no one will even notice—but a step in the raw direction.

OPTION 2: To make it a little more raw, substitute 100% whole spelt, kamut, or brown rice pasta for your standard white or whole-wheat. This is a step toward breaking your dependency on wheat.

OPTION 3: To make the sauce raw, put chopped raw tomatoes in the blender, add cold-pressed olive oil and sea salt, and blend. Pour the sauce over the hot pasta to heat up the tomato sauce— the tomato sauce will be warm, but still raw. Bonus for heartburn sufferers: By not cooking your tomatoes, you might find yourself free of the burn at the end of this meal.

totally raw pasta with tomato sauce

For the pasta, substitute raw squash pasta cut from a spiral slicer (see page 30) for the wheat pasta, and make your tomato sauce raw, as described in Option 3, above. All raw—well done!

AMERICA'S FAVORITE SANDWICH IN THE RAW

For a partially raw sandwich, take two slices of Ezekiel bread, spread one side with raw nut butter (see recipe, page 100) and the other with raw dried fruit jam (see recipe, page 101), press together, and eat. For a fully raw sandwich, choose a bread recipe from pages 220 to 221 or a packaged bread from the Sources section (page 239).

seventeen ways to add a little raw to your meals

1. Add your cold-pressed oil and sea salt at the end of the cooking time whenever you can.

2. Keep your pantry supplied with all the makings of a raw salad dressing: cold-pressed oils and raw apple cider vinegar or coconut vinegar.

3. Use sprouted chickpeas (see page 39) instead of cooked chickpeas in your salad.

4. Use fresh vegetables instead of canned.

5. Use kefir (see page 50) instead of yogurt or pasteurized juices in your smoothies.

6. Use raw dairy milk or a nut milk (see recipe, page 88) on your cooked cereal or pasteurized milk on your raw cereal to make your breakfast about half raw.

7. Buy unsweetened frozen fruits rather than fruits packed in syrup.

8. Choose a sprouted grain (see page 36) rather than a cooked grain to serve with your meal or in your salad.

9. Freeze your own vegetables, such as tomatoes, corn, and peas (packaged frozen foods are blanched—briefly boiled—before freezing).

10. For vegetable soup, bring your soup stock to boil, add your raw vegetables, and remove from the heat. Give them time to soften rather than cooking them.

11. Order unpasteurized almonds and raw agave nectar online (see Sources, page 239) in bulk so you always have some around for recipes and snacking.

12. Buy raw rather than roasted nuts in the bulk section of your supermarket—most stores will have both.

13. Create your own trail mix with raw nuts and dehydrated packaged fruits, or make your own dehydrated fruit (see page 40).

14. Substitute rapadura (pure brown sugar; see page 52) for white sugar in your coffee or tea.

15. Make just one meal of your day raw—breakfast is an easy one to start with.

16. Make your sandwiches with raw cheeses, gravlax (salt-cured fish; see recipe, page 154), or prosciutto (salt-cured and air-dried pork) instead of the usual cold cuts.

17. Sear your meat or fish so it is a little cooked on the outside but raw on the inside.

perfectly seared steak with potatoes

If you're a meat eater, you may not wish to go totally raw in the meat department. Carpaccio (raw beef) isn't for everyone—that's understandable. But that doesn't mean that you have to go to the other extreme and cook the life out of your steak. The happy medium is to sear your steak—briefly cook it over high heat so it's slightly cooked on the outside and uncooked on the inside, maximizing flavor and keeping it partially raw. Before you buy the beef, please make sure it's grass-fed or tell your butcher that you will be lightly searing your meat. (Note that many restaurants will do a "black and blue"— I recommend asking for a "brown and blue.")

cooked steak with mashed potatoes

Cook your steak through until no pink remains and serve with dairy mashed potatoes.

partially raw steak with mashed potatoes

Sear your steak and cook it to medium-rare. Boil your potatoes and mash them, adding cold-pressed extra-virgin olive oil and sea salt at the end.

¾ to 1 pound organic grass-fed beef steak

1 teaspoon freshly ground black pepper

1 teaspoon dried herbs, such as rosemary, thyme, or oregano (or a mixture), optional

½ teaspoon sea salt

Must-Have Mustard (page 105) or Mayonnaise (page 104), for serving (optional)

Garlicky Salt and Vinegar Potato Chips (page 226)

as raw as you like it steak with garlicky salt and vinegar potato chips

{ SERVES 2 }

What I am trying to do with these recipes is teach you how to eat healthier and enjoy food, so make your steak as raw as you feel comfortable with. Serve with one of my salad recipes for a completely balanced meal.

Pat the beef dry and season with the pepper and herbs, if using, massaging the mixture into the surface of the meat to evenly coat. Let sit for 30 minutes before cooking.

Heat a large cast-iron skillet over high heat until very hot. Place the meat in the pan and sear to desired doneness, for a few seconds or up to 2 minutes on each side. Place on a cutting board, let rest for a couple of minutes, and then slice and divide between two plates. Season with the salt. Serve with some mustard or mayonnaise and, if you like, with the chips.

A PATTERN TO PRESERVING RAW-NESS

Do you see a pattern here? Adding oils, salts, and flavorings after you remove food from the heat will preserve their rawness. Use what you've learned so far and start turning *your* favorite recipes raw: There are so many ingredients that can be added like this at the last minute, putting you ahead of the game on the road to raw.

chocolate chocolate chip cookies

Even cookies can go raw, and I guarantee you will love raw cookies every bit as much as their cooked counterparts. To make your cookies either partially or totally raw, you'll need a dehydrator and a little bit of patience, as they take 8 to 10 hours to dehydrate (plus soaking time for the nuts). But the reward is worth the wait.

cooked chocolate chocolate chip cookies

Mix up all your ingredients and bake. Even if you start out with raw chocolate, sweeteners, and the like, once your cookies spend some time in the oven, they are 100 percent cooked.

partially raw chocolate chocolate chip cookies

Haven't ordered your raw almonds online yet (see Sources, page 239)? Follow the totally raw recipe opposite but use store-bought (pasteurized) almonds, regular cacao powder, and/or a regular chocolate bar.

1½ cups raw almonds, soaked (see page 38)

1 cup raw walnuts, soaked (see page 38)

1 packed cup halved and pitted Medjool dates, soaked in water for about 30 minutes, and roughly chopped

¼ cup raw cacao powder

¼ cup raw honey or raw agave nectar

1 teaspoon alcohol-free vanilla extract

¼ teaspoon sea salt

One 3-ounce raw chocolate bar (see Sources, page 239), finely chopped

totally raw chocolate chocolate chip cookies

{ MAKES ABOUT 2 DOZEN COOKIES }

You might want to double the recipe so you always have dessert at the ready. If you are not a fan of chocolate, omit the cacao powder and chocolate bar for a simple but equally delicious cookie—one that's so healthy you could eat it for breakfast!

Combine all the ingredients except the chocolate bar in a food processor and process until they start to form a ball, scraping the sides of the bowl a few times (you may need to do this in 2 batches). Transfer to a bowl and add the chopped chocolate, using your clean hands to work the chips in.

Using a small cookie scoop about 1½ inches in diameter, scoop up the batter and place the mounds on a mesh screen–lined dehydrator tray and place in the dehydrator. Set the machine to 115°F and dehydrate for 12 to 16 hours, until firm on the outside but still a little moist on the inside. Eat a few warm from the dehydrator! Cool the rest and store in an airtight container in the refrigerator for up to 2 weeks or in the freezer for up to 2 months.

{ variation }

BITE-SIZE COOKIES: Use a very small cookie scoop, about 1 inch in diameter, to form the dough and dehydrate for the same amount of time; the yield will be about 6 dozen cookies.

seven tips for turning it raw in restaurants

1. Bring your own salad dressing (see page 123).

2. Request a special-order salad as your main dish.

3. Ask to substitute a salad for cooked vegetable sides.

4. Order your fish or steak lightly seared—so it's cooked on the outside but still raw on the inside.

5. In Japanese restaurants, choose sashimi (raw fish without rice) rather than sushi.

6. In Indian restaurants, order dosas (rice and lentil crêpes). The crêpes are cooked, but the batter is fermented, and the chutneys that come with it are more likely to be raw than anything else on the menu.

7. In Thai and Vietnamese restaurants, choose raw vegetable–based starters such as mango salad or papaya salad and take advantage of the generous amount of fresh ingredients, such as shallots, cilantro, mint, and basil, that typically come with soups and other dishes.

breakfast like a king

At the turn of the twentieth century, many people in the United States started their day with a version of this breakfast: bacon, potatoes, biscuits, eggs, pork chops, and cheese. A few years later? They ate cereal.

What happened? Kellogg's introduced an easy breakfast for those on the go—and it was the dawning of a new world. But the fact is, you do need a substantial breakfast to fuel your day. Eat cold cooked cereal and inevitably you'll be reaching for that snack at eleven a.m. Or eating a big dinner at night.

Once you start to favor real food, your taste buds will begin to wake up ready for action. So let's make those taste buds happy with my raw breakfast recipes.

basic smoothie

1½ to 2 cups liquid such as water, coconut water, raw dairy milk, Basic Nut or Seed Milk (page 88), Basic Kefir (page 90), or fresh-squeezed orange juice

1 frozen sliced banana

½ cup frozen berries (see tip) or other fruit

optional ingredients

1 tablespoon flax oil or Udo's Choice Oil Blend

1 tablespoon hemp seeds, flax seeds, or chia seeds

1 to 2 tablespoons green (spirulina) powder

1 Medjool date, halved and pitted, or a little raw honey, raw agave nectar, coconut nectar, rapadura, or stevia if you like it sweeter

My boyfriend is a smoothie junkie, and he has sort of forced me into being a smoothie genius! He doesn't like commercial smoothie joints, because many of them go a little crazy with the add-ins: Ingredients such as pasteurized milk, low-quality sweeteners, syrup, and sometimes even ice cream may make it into your drink! That's when your smoothie becomes a high-calorie dessert in a glass, rather than a good-for-you start to the day.

When you make a smoothie with fruit, it satisfies the sweet tooth naturally (but don't go overboard on the fruit or, again, it's dessert). And when you freeze your fruit before blending, it makes your smoothie creamy, just as if you had added ice cream.

Stock your freezer with bags of frozen fruit (make sure they aren't in syrup) from the supermarket, and cut up some bananas and freeze them so you always have some around. Then blend with your beverage of choice and whatever extras you like, and you're good to go. The following is my standard smoothie recipe—use it as a base, mix it up, and you'll never drink the same smoothie twice.

....

In a blender, combine all the ingredients and blend until smooth. Serve immediately.

{ variations }

GREEN SMOOTHIE: Add a handful of leafy greens, such as kale, spinach, or lettuce. Add ½ beet, peeled and chopped, to offset the green color and give yourself a boost of iron.

SUPER-CREAMY SMOOTHIE: Add ½ avocado or ¼ cup young coconut meat.

NUTTY SMOOTHIE: Add 1 tablespoon Nutty Butter (page 100).

POMEGRANATE SMOOTHIE: Add the seeds of ½ pomegranate.

CRANBERRY-ORANGE SMOOTHIE: Use cranberries in place of the berries and orange juice for your liquid.

tip

To keep your berries perfectly whole when you freeze them, spread them on a baking sheet in a single layer and freeze for about 1 hour, until solid. Then transfer to a freezer bag or plastic container and return to the freezer.

When you juice, you're getting a straight shot of vitamins and minerals—your body just takes them in and absorbs them, with nothing standing in their way (see pages 45 and 46 for more on the benefits of juicing). When you make a smoothie, the pulp is retained, so you get an added hit of fiber. It takes longer to digest than a juice, and it can be a little more stabilizing for your body.

CINNAMON-APPLE SMOOTHIE: Use apple in place of the berries and add a pinch of ground cinnamon.

GOJI SMOOTHIE: Add a handful of goji berries.

PUMPKIN PIE SMOOTHIE: Substitute grated pumpkin or winter squash for the berries and add a pinch each of cinnamon, ginger, and nutmeg.

TROPICAL SMOOTHIE: Use papaya in place of the berries and add a tablespoon of dried coconut.

starving for fats

You can be a skinny size 2, a plus size, or anywhere in between and still be dehydrated and starving—not for water but for fats. What does that feel like? You'll eat, and you won't be satisfied. So you'll start eating more. Or you'll always feel hungry and deprived.

That was me when I first went raw. I consulted with my doctor, and my prescription was so rich in fats, I couldn't believe it was doctor's orders. I don't need quite so much fat now, but back then, coming off the fat-is-bad-for-you mentality, I sure did.

My daily morning drink would be made up of young coconut, raw butter, raw milk, green powder, coconut water, raw honey, and avocado. The first time my doctor made it for me, I had to get past the avocado (guacamole for breakfast?). But once I took that leap of faith, I gulped it down in seconds. I had four cups, then I licked the blender. I was in fat heaven.

My doctor encouraged me to drink up, because my body was literally starving for essential fatty acids. The drink worked to trade in my tired old fats for clean, raw fats and rebuild my body, storing the rest for later so I wouldn't always be running on empty.

Fat free I wasn't, but I never gained an ounce. And all of a sudden I wasn't tired and hungry all the time, like I was when I was a model.

lucuma smoothie

1 cup raw dairy milk or
Basic Nut or Seed Milk
(page 88)

3 to 4 tablespoons
lucuma powder

2 tablespoons raw
honey, raw agave
nectar, or rapadura

1 teaspoon alcohol-free
vanilla extract

Handful of ice cubes

Ever hear of lucuma? No, it's not a disease! It's a fragrant tropical fruit hailing from Peru; there it makes its way into many recipes, ice cream being one of the most popular. Because of its nutritional properties and slightly sweet taste, in recent years raw foodists have discovered it in a big way, adding it to smoothies, raw ice cream, puddings, and the like.

Though fresh lucuma in this part of the world is a rarity, the powder, bright yellow in color, can be ordered in its raw state online (see Sources, page 239). This healthy fruit is filled with vitamins and minerals, and it imparts a light butterscotch flavor and a creamy texture to smoothies. You can also sprinkle it on top of Raw Granola (page 81), Prune and Chia Porridge (opposite), or any other breakfast cereal in place of honey or agave nectar.

In a blender, combine all the ingredients and blend until smooth. Serve immediately.

{ variation }

CHOCOLATE LUCUMA SMOOTHIE: Add 1 tablespoon raw cacao powder.

keeping raw milk on hand

Freeze raw milk so you always have some on hand for your smoothies, and keep it in single-serving portions so you only need to defrost one for each smoothie. If you happen to have a silicone muffin pan from your baking days, it will come in handy as a milk holder: Place it on a baking sheet, fill the cups with milk, and freeze for about 2 hours, until solid. Then pop the individual portions of milk into a freezer bag for storage and return to the freezer. Alternatively, freeze your milk in ice cube trays.

prune and chia porridge

{ SERVES 2 TO 3 }

¼ to ½ cup pitted prunes

1 to 2 tablespoons raw honey, raw agave nectar, coconut nectar, or rapadura

½ cup raw almonds, cashews, soaked (see page 38) or raw macadamia nuts soaked in water to cover for 1 hour

1 teaspoon alcohol-free vanilla extract, or ¼ teaspoon alcohol-free almond extract

Dash of sea salt

½ cup chia seeds

timesaver
Make the cereal the night before and you'll have no morning prep.

ALMOST YOGURT

Add a teaspoon or so of chia seeds to your milk, stir, and let sit for about 30 minutes; it will thicken like yogurt.

Yes, it's those chia seeds, of Chia Pet fame. They may be good for a bit of fun, but the amount of nutrition that's packed into each seed is no joke! They are an excellent source of calcium, iron, protein, fiber, and omega-3 fatty acids, among other nutrients. A superfood that will make you feel like a supermodel!

And chia seeds are wonderfully versatile: When you add water to them, they swell up and thicken, making them the perfect ingredient to use in raw puddings and porridge, like this rich, nutty tasting breakfast treat. Or add a spoonful to your smoothie to thicken it, use as a topping for Raw Granola (page 81) or Pass the Buck Cereal (page 80), or sprinkle over Just Bananas Pancakes (page 82).

In a blender, blend 2 cups water with all the ingredients except the chia seeds.

Place the chia seeds in a bowl or container, pour the prune mixture over them, and mix well to coat all the seeds. Cover and refrigerate for at least 30 minutes to soften.

{ variation }

PRUNE AND CARDAMOM CHIA PORRIDGE: Substitute ¼ teaspoon ground cardamom for the vanilla.

almost instant chia porridge
Follow this simple formula for a version of chia porridge that can be put together in minutes: For one serving, combine ¼ cup chia seeds and 1 cup water, stir, set aside for 30 minutes, then add your choice of milk, fruit, and/or raw sweetener.

pass the buck cereal

{ SERVES 4 TO 6 }

6 cups sprouted buckwheat (see page 39)

Often called buckwheaties in the raw world, this breakfast cereal takes a bit of advance planning—it involves soaking, sprouting, and dehydrating. But don't let that scare you away—it only requires one ingredient! And it keeps for a few weeks, so you can double or triple the recipe—fill up all the trays of your dehydrator—and have it on hand whenever you get the urge for something a little crunchy.

Make sure you use hulled raw buckwheat groats, which are a whitish green to light brown color, and not kasha. A little darker in color, kasha is toasted, which means it won't sprout.

A note on soaking: Buckwheat groats release a large amount of starch when they are soaked, so make sure to rinse the buckwheat well both before and after soaking to remove some of the starch. You won't be able to remove it all, but that's fine.

Spread out the sprouted buckwheat on ParaFlexx-lined dehydrator trays. Place in the dehydrator, set it for 115°F, and dehydrate for 10 to 12 hours, until crisp. Serve with your choice of milk, fruit, and/or sweetener.

Store in an airtight container for up to 3 weeks.

---

buckwheat is wheat free

Good news for those who are avoiding wheat: Despite its misleading name, buckwheat has no relation to wheat and is completely gluten free.

raw granola

{ SERVES 1 }

½ cup your choice of raw nuts and/or seeds, soaked (see pages 38–39)

2 tablespoons sprouted oat groats (see page 39)

1 or 2 Medjool dates, halved and pitted

COMFORT FOOD FOR FALL

Add a little cinnamon and a drizzle of coconut nectar—coconut nectar has a deep, molasses flavor— with warm milk for a fulfilling brisk-weather breakfast.

This granola fills you up but won't weigh you down, unlike the sugar-laden cooked granola you get at the supermarket, which would be more appropriately placed in the candy aisle than the breakfast cereal aisle.

This is not so much a recipe as a guideline for a great simple breakfast—go ahead and make it with whatever ingredients call to you when you open the cupboard in the morning (bananas always call to me). You don't really even have to measure—a little of this, a little of that, and as simple or fancy as you like.

....

Combine the soaked nuts, sprouted oats, and date in a food processor and pulse until you have a very coarse puree. Add your choice of flavorings, if you like:

    ¼ teaspoon alcohol-free vanilla extract, or a couple of drops of alcohol-free almond extract

    ¼ teaspoon ground cinnamon, or a pinch of ground nutmeg, cloves, or allspice

Then pour over some raw dairy milk or choice of Basic Nut or Seed Milk (page 88); warm the milk slightly first if you like.

    Add a topping or two, such as:

Grated fresh or dried shredded coconut

Raisins

Goji berries

Sliced bananas or whole berries

A drizzle of raw honey, agave nectar, or coconut nectar, or a sprinkle of rapadura

just bananas pancakes

4 large ripe bananas

⅓ cup ground chia seeds (grind them in a coffee grinder or buy them preground)

1 teaspoon alcohol-free vanilla extract

Hold the honey till you taste them. These pancakes come with their own natural sweetener inside: bananas. This recipe is the perfect example of how easy preparing raw foods can be: Blend up the batter just before you go to bed, place in the dehydrator, and breakfast is ready when you wake up in the morning.

Serve with Applesauce (page 103), a fresh fruit of your choosing, a little Dairy Whipped Cream Topping (page 198), or a sweetener if you are so inclined.

In a high-speed blender or food processor, combine all the ingredients and blend until smooth, pressing down with the tamper as you blend if using a Vitamix, or scraping the sides once or twice if using a food processor.

Using a ¼-cup measure, drop 8 mounds of the batter onto ParaFlexx sheets. Form them into pancake shapes that are about 3 inches in diameter and ½ inch thick (you will be using 2 sheets). Place on dehydrator trays and place in the dehydrator. Turn it to 115°F and dehydrate for 8 hours, until the pancakes are fairly firm on the sides and soft in the middle (they don't need to be solid like cooked pancakes).

HOW TO MAKE PERFECTLY ROUND RAW PANCAKES

When you cook pancakes, the heat of the pan moves the batter around and does the work of forming a circle for you. Since you don't have that heat, try this trick: Scoop the batter with a flat-bottom ¼-cup measure, pour the batter onto your ParaFlexx sheets in mounds, and gently rotate the bottom of the measuring cup over each mound to form a perfect circle.

{ variations }

CINNAMON-RAISIN PANCAKES: Add ⅓ cup coarsely chopped raisins and ½ teaspoon ground cinnamon to the batter.

CHOCOLATE PANCAKES: Add 2 tablespoons raw cacao powder to the batter.

SILVER DOLLAR PANCAKES: Use heaping tablespoonfuls of batter to form small pancakes, about 20 pancakes that are 1½ inches wide and ½ inch thick.

coco-mango pancakes

4 large ripe bananas

⅓ cup dried shredded coconut

⅓ cup ground chia seeds (grind them in a coffee grinder or buy them preground)

1 teaspoon alcohol-free vanilla extract

4 dried mango pieces, chopped (see Note)

¼ cup finely chopped raw macadamia nuts

This is a version of my banana pancakes gone tropical, and filled with lots of healthy fats from the coconut and macadamias to jump-start your day.

In a high-speed blender or food processor, combine the bananas, coconut, chia seeds, and vanilla and blend until smooth, pressing down with the tamper as you blend if using a Vitamix, or scraping the sides once or twice if using a food processor. Add the mango pieces and pulse until blended in, with a few bits remaining. Stir in the macadamias.

Using a ¼-cup measure, drop 8 mounds of the batter onto ParaFlexx sheets. Form them into pancake shapes that are about 3 inches in diameter and ½ inch thick (you will be using 2 sheets). Place on dehydrator trays and place in the dehydrator. Turn it to 115°F and dehydrate for 8 hours, until the pancakes are fairly firm on the sides and soft in the middle (they don't need to be solid like cooked pancakes).

NOTE: If your dried mangos are too stiff to chop, soak them in warm water for 30 minutes before using.

on-the-go cranberry-nut breakfast bars

{ **MAKES 1 DOZEN BARS** }

2 cups raw almonds, soaked (see page 38)

½ cup hemp seeds

½ cup flax or chia seeds

¼ teaspoon sea salt

1 cup halved and pitted Medjool dates

2 cups fresh cranberries

½ cup raw honey

FLIP IT AND SCORE IT

To flip your dehydrator goodies, place an empty ParaFlexx-lined dehydrator tray over what you're making, then turn the whole thing upside down and remove the top sheet.

Then score with a butter knife in the shape of the finished bars, so they will be easier to separate when done.

I never sit still—why would I? Big world, lots to do! So I grab one of these bars to go any time of day, whether I'm on the set, at my office, or on the trail—whenever I'm looking for an energy boost. They will need 24 hours in the dehydrator, but the good news is that the prep time is minimal.

Drain the almonds, place them in a food processor, and grind them until they form a thick paste, with some bits remaining, scraping the sides of the machine once or twice. Transfer to a large bowl and add the hemp seeds, flax seeds, and salt.

Place the dates in the food processor, add 2 tablespoons water, and process to a puree.

In a medium bowl, toss the cranberries with the honey until coated. Add to the dates in the food processor and pulse until pureed, with a few chunks remaining. Transfer the puree to the bowl with the seeds and mix well.

Spread out the mixture on a ParaFlexx sheet so that it's about 12 inches wide and ½ inch thick (it will cover most of the sheet). Place the sheet on a dehydrator tray and place in the dehydrator. Set it to 105°F and dehydrate for 12 hours. Flip the whole thing, score it into 12 bars, and dehydrate for an additional 12 hours, until firm and slightly crisp, but still soft inside.

{ variation }

CRANBERRY-NUT CEREAL: Break the bars into bits to turn them into a breakfast cereal. For a soft cereal, dehydrate for only 12 hours.

drink up

Who doesn't like a cool drink on a warm day or a warm drink on a cold day?

Whether it's to quench your thirst, nourish your body, or for the enjoyment of it all, these recipes—from a centuries-old sports drink to homemade soft drinks and the wonderful probiotic beverage kefir— won't disappoint. So drop the sugary beverage and step away from the table. Enjoy these healthier versions of your favorite drinks! And if you're wondering about alcohol and raw, see page 86 for some thoughts on the subject.

listen to the doctor:
the scoop on alcohol

When people meet me for the first time, the inevitable first question, "What do you eat?" is often followed by "Do you drink alcohol?"

Now I know that drinking is a social pastime, but based on my research and a discussion with an expert on the subject, I believe that it may not be such a good idea to drink.

First of all, it ages you. So you spend your money on the wine, and then on the plastic surgery! How does it age you? In my own words: Alcohol swings the system acidic; acidity causes inflammation, and inflammation leads to disease. The way I picture this, to use a somewhat graphic analogy: Acid is like rust on your car; it eats the body from the inside out. The body knows this and tries to balance this acid by using its store of minerals. (How it does this is a complex scientific process, so here I'll just say it uses important youth-maintaining minerals to do it, thereby, as the saying goes, "wasting your youth.")

Second, and most important, is that I find I crave alcohol when I am hungry. Irish coffee used to be my big thing; I craved it because I was always dieting. Now that I eat raw, I find that for the most part I don't even want, can't even look at, can't even stand the smell of alcohol. And if I do have a hankering for it, it is a sign to me that I have not eaten correctly that day. After I eat well, the craving usually goes away.

But don't just listen to me. Listen to the doctor—Dr. Richard Firshein, doctor to the stars and author of *The Vitamin Prescription* (2010), *The Neutraceutical Revolution* (1998), and *Reversing Asthma* (1996). The information on diet in *Reversing Asthma* saved the doctor's own life—kind of the same thing I am trying to do here for you! Here's what Dr. Firshein told me about alcohol and its effects on the liver:

The liver is the second-largest organ in our body, after our skin. It has the unique capacity to monitor and affect almost every biochemical process in the body. If the substance is a toxin, such as alcohol, the liver will break it down and make it "biodegradable" so that it can be eliminated as waste. But only up to a point.

Because of the increasing amounts of toxins that we are constantly exposing ourselves to, our livers are completely overworked and overloaded. Once the liver's workload becomes more than it can handle, the result is a higher level of toxicity in the body, ultimately compromising our health. The toxins build up quickly with alcohol. Once the liver's workload is exceeded, the harmful effects of alcohol start to appear.

So what exactly happens when you have that martini or glass of wine? About 25 percent of the alcohol enters the bloodstream from your stomach and the rest is mostly absorbed by blood vessels in your small intestine. The alcohol in your bloodstream is carried throughout your body until it is processed. Then between 90 and 98 percent is excreted by the liver. The other 2 to 10 percent of alcohol is removed in your urine, breath, or sweat.

Our livers process alcohol in two phases:

Phase I: During a process called bioactivation, your body's liver enzymes may "activate" certain compounds, which can increase systemic toxicity.

Phase II: The more dangerous toxins that were too stubborn to be eliminated in Phase I are converted into more water-soluble forms, which your body eliminates through urine or stool. Partially processed toxins are not easily eliminated and instead pass from the liver back into the body—and there is the problem! (The body's natural inclination is, of course, to get rid of toxins, but when the system gets overloaded as a result of unhealthy foods, alcohol, and so on, it cannot remove them all.)

If these toxins are not removed, eventually they are stored in fatty tissue, the central nervous system, and even in our joints. About 90 percent of all degenerative diseases are thought to be caused by a dysfunctional or overstressed liver because the liver affects so many body systems. Ultimately this all speeds up the aging process. It also contributes to the significant increase in cancer and chronic illnesses. When these toxins are produced and/or not eliminated, they lead to an acidic environment in the body, which contributes to many disease states. (My point exactly!)

But don't fret—if you have been drinking alcohol and want to soothe your liver, there is some help available. The doctor recommends:

- Favoring foods that have a powerful supportive effect on the liver, including raw garlic and onions, cruciferous vegetables (broccoli, cauliflower, Brussels sprouts, cabbage), whole grains, berries, green tea, legumes, nuts and seeds, red grapes, and turmeric.

- Reducing your intake of processed and preserved foods (eat raw, eat raw!), and limit your consumption of alcohol, coffee, soft drinks, and refined sugar.

- Looking into nutritional supplements and juicing. Herbal remedies such as milk thistle, dandelion root, and burdock root and the amino acids N-Acetyl Cysteine (NAC) and taurine have proven to be very potent liver-protecting agents, which can serve as a counterbalance to alcohol. (But don't take this as license to go ahead and drink with abandon!) Consult with your health-care provider to choose the supplements that work best for you.

basic nut or seed milk

1 cup raw nuts or seeds, soaked (see pages 38–39)

1 teaspoon alcohol-free vanilla extract, or ¼ teaspoon alcohol-free almond extract (optional)

1 tablespoon raw honey or agave nectar, or 1 or 2 Medjool dates, pitted (optional)

NUT MILK THE CHEATER'S WAY

Combine some water, raw almond butter, and a little honey. Blend, and voilà—nut milk the cheater's way!

Afraid of raw milk? Can't find it? Don't get frustrated—nut milk is your answer. It is indispensable in the raw kitchen, particularly if you're dairy free. You can use it any way you would use dairy milk: on your cereal—I love it on my raw granola (page 81)—in smoothies, as a base for soup, or as a tasty drink on its own.

The boxes of nut milk you find on natural foods store shelves are not raw—even if they're labeled "organic." For nut milk to be shelf stable, it has to be cooked. And some brands are sweetened with sugar and contain other non-raw flavoring ingredients to boot. Luckily, if you keep a supply of soaked nuts on hand, it's a breeze to make your own, and it costs a lot less, too.

Almond milk is my favorite, but you can use just about any type of nut or seed—cashews, Brazil nuts, sunflower seeds, sesame seeds, and even hemp seeds. Use the lesser amount of water for a thicker nut milk, and the greater amount for a thinner nut milk, and sweeten it to your liking. It will keep in the refrigerator in an airtight container for about 4 days.

In a high-speed blender, combine the nuts with 3 to 5 cups water and blend until the nuts are ground to a pulp. Strain through a fine-mesh strainer lined with cheesecloth or through a nut milk bag (see Sources, page 239) and press or squeeze out all the liquid. Reserve the nut pulp for another use (add it to your raw granola for a creamy porridge). Add the vanilla and honey if using.

health is wealth turmeric milk

{ **SERVES 1** }

1 tablespoon raw pistachios

1 cup raw dairy milk or Basic Nut or Seed milk (opposite)

¼ teaspoon ground turmeric

2 teaspoons raw honey, or to taste

Pinch of saffron threads

As I mentioned earlier, before I went raw, my life was all about pills—pills for my digestion, pills for the colds I was always getting, and pills to fall asleep. I could have used a good shot of turmeric milk back then.

This tried-and-true healing beverage from India is good for what ails you, from settling your stomach, to treating a cold, to helping you sleep. It's comfort food in a glass, and there's science to back up these claims: The active ingredient in turmeric, curcumin, has been found to work as an antiinflammatory and can reduce fever and aches, without the side effects of over-the-counter drugs. Try a cup just before bed for a restful sleep.

In a coffee grinder, grind the pistachios to a powder.

Pour the milk into a small saucepan. Place over medium heat and heat until just warm to the touch or, if you have an instant-read thermometer, until the milk reaches 110°F.

One at a time, whisk in the turmeric, honey, and pistachio powder until dissolved. Pour into a mug and crumble the saffron on top.

---

timesaver
If you are making turmeric milk a regular bedtime drink, grind up a week's worth of pistachios at a time so you'll have them at the ready.

basic kefir

2 tablespoons kefir starter

2 cups raw dairy milk

COCONUT KEFIR

You can make kefir out of young coconut water, too. Here's how: Heat the coconut water on the stovetop until warm to the touch, or, if you have an instant-read thermometer, until it reaches 92°F. Pour it into a glass container, add kefir cultures as you would for dairy kefir, put the lid on, and shake well. Leave at room temperature for about 36 hours, until cloudy and lighter in color. The resulting kefir will have a slightly tangy taste with a little fizz, but it will not thicken like dairy kefir. It will keep for about a week in the refrigerator.

I was never really crazy about yogurt, but kefir is just plain mm mm good. That's why earlier in the book (see page 50) I talked your ear off about the benefits of this amazing probiotic drink that makes nutritional magic out of milk. Here I will show you the step-by-step method for preparing it at home. The recipe is infinitely expandable. You'll need 1 tablespoon of kefir starter per cup of milk.

So many people tell me they are confused by the kefir starter (also called a grain, culture, or bud), so let me explain. It is made of the kefir itself and looks like a tiny cauliflower. The starter ferments the milk, incorporating its beneficial bacteria. Then the liquid is strained and drunk, and you start the process over again for the next batch, using the original grain and fresh milk. If properly cared for, the starter can last a lifetime, and over time it multiplies, so you can share it with your friends! GEM Cultures (see Sources, page 239) is a reliable mail-order source for kefir starters.

1. Place the kefir starter in a glass jar, and pour the milk over it.

2. Cover the jar loosely and set aside on the counter where it will be out of direct sunlight for 12 to 24 hours, stirring occasionally, until thickened. Do not refrigerate. The longer it sits, the thicker and tangier it gets—experiment to see how you like it.

3. Strain the liquid kefir into a glass or pitcher, reserving the leftover starter. Drink the liquid, or cover and refrigerate for up to a week.

4. Place the starter back in the original jar and start the process over again. Wash the jar every third batch or so.

KEFIR WITHOUT THE CLEANUP

If you're keen on making kefir but don't have the time for straining, the Body Ecology and Yógourmet kefir starter kits are good alternatives (see Sources, page 239).

The starters come in the form of a powder, making them great for travel. You simply mix the powder into the milk, leave it to ferment, and your kefir is ready; no straining necessary. You do pay a price for that convenience, though, as the starter lasts for several batches rather than forever like the traditional kefir cultures. But if it gets you to drink kefir, in my opinion, that's a small price to pay!

tips for making and keeping kefir

- If your kefir is made but you're not ready to drink it, refrigerate it, loosely covered, with the starter still in it, until you're ready to strain and drink it. It will keep for a couple of weeks. Refrigeration greatly slows down the fermentation process. This is a good option for vacations or breaks from kefir.

- If you're out of milk, you can keep the kefir starter submerged in water in the refrigerator for a few days until you're ready to make your next batch.

- If your kefir drink goes bad while you're making it, strain the starter and wash it well. No need to replace the starter, as the starter itself won't go bad.

- Your kefir starter will multiply as you continue to make your batches; share the kefir "babies" with friends and family.

NOTE: Don't freak out if you think kefir is too difficult or time-consuming to make. You just may not have the time to make kefir this week.

So allow me to introduce the Lazy Man's Kefir: Just take a spoonful of your finished kefir or a portion of your kefir grains and freeze it. This will be the bud for your next kefir whenever the laziness or busyness passes. Freezing doesn't destroy the bacteria; it just stops its action until it is thawed.

Usually I leave about a tablespoon of finished kefir in the jar I made it in and freeze it, jar and all. My frozen container becomes my backup plan in case the bacteria doesn't take in a later batch for some reason. This can happen to anyone, so don't fret or feel lame if you get a batch that doesn't produce kefir. Just go to your backup frozen bacteria, thaw it, and you are ready to start a new batch.

lassis

Lassi is a yogurt drink found on the menu of every Indian restaurant. I make my "live" version with kefir, which gives it a tangy edge and a hefty dose of friendly probiotic cultures.

Mango is the most popular lassi flavor. I've also included recipes for an exotic rosewater lassi and a traditional, refreshing salt lassi (yes, salt can actually be refreshing—a billion Indians can attest to it!) for the hot days of summer.

rosewater lassi

1 cup Basic Kefir (page 90)

2 tablespoons raw honey or raw agave nectar, or to taste

1 tablespoon rosewater

{ SERVES 1 }

Pour the kefir into a glass, add the honey and rosewater, and stir to dissolve. Serve over ice if you like.

salt lassi

1 cup Basic Kefir (page 90)

2 pinches of sea salt, or to taste

2 pinches of ground cumin

Handful of chopped fresh cilantro or mint leaves

{ SERVES 1 }

Pour the kefir into a glass, add the salt and cumin, and stir to dissolve. Add the cilantro or mint and serve over ice if you like.

mango lassi

1 cup Basic Kefir (page 90)

1 mango, peeled, flesh cut away from the pit, and chopped

Pinch of ground cardamom

1 tablespoon raw honey or raw agave nectar, or to taste

Pinch of saffron threads

{ SERVES 1 }

Combine all the ingredients in a blender and blend until smooth. Pour into a glass. Serve over ice if you like.

ginger ale

{ SERVES 1 OR 2 }

1 to 2 teaspoons ginger juice (see below)

1 teaspoon fresh lime juice, or to taste

3 to 4 tablespoons raw agave nectar

Small pinch of sea salt

2 cups sparkling water

---

timesaver

If you're a big ginger ale drinker, juice a week's worth of ginger at a time and store in the refrigerator.

There's something not quite right in the world when you see commercial soft drink packaging boasting "made with real sugar." Folks, sugar isn't a health food, even if the alternative they've been using for the past few decades—high-fructose corn syrup—is nothing to brag about.

Another curious fact: Most commercial ginger ales don't contain real ginger, even if they happen to contain real sugar! Sidestep the whole issue and make your own: This recipe is the real deal.

....

In a small pitcher, combine the ginger juice, lime juice, agave, and salt. Add the sparkling water and quickly stir until the ingredients are combined. Pour into glasses and drink immediately.

{ variation }

Add a splash of your favorite raw juice—cranberry, apple, orange, whatever you like.

FOUR WAYS TO JUICE GINGER

1. Finely grate the ginger (no need to peel it first) and squeeze it between your fingers to extract the juice. If you like, wrap the ginger in cheesecloth to make straining easier. Ginger freezes well; you can store a few pieces to have on hand whenever a recipe calls for it. It's not necessary to thaw it before grating—it's actually easier to grate when it's frozen.

2. Run the ginger through a juicer: a good option when you are making a lot of juice or when you've already got the juicer out to make your morning vegetable juice (juice the ginger before the green veggies).

3. Pass small pieces of ginger through a garlic press.

4. Use a ceramic ginger grater: This dedicated tool has sharp teeth, which you run the ginger over. It extracts the juice and leaves the fiber behind.

summer coolers

I'm not an air-conditioning person—I prefer the heat. So I need to keep myself cool but raw, and these two drinks are not only raw but practically calorie free (not that you have to worry much about calories when you go raw, but it can't hurt). Some people find stevia to be cloyingly sweet, but I've found that it works well in tangy or tart drinks like these, as the sour citrus balances the intense sweetness of the stevia. You can find dried hibiscus flowers in herb shops and Mexican and Caribbean groceries.

hibiscus lemonade

1 tablespoon plus
1 teaspoon dried
hibiscus flowers

4 cups warm water

Juice of 1 lemon
(about 3 tablespoons),
or to taste

25 drops liquid stevia,
or to taste

{ MAKES 1 QUART }

Place the hibiscus in a large bowl, add the 4 cups warm water, and steep for 1 hour. Strain the hibiscus tea into a glass pitcher. Add the lemon juice and stevia and stir. Add more lemon juice or stevia to taste if you like. Refrigerate until cold, and serve over ice.

tamarind water

1 tablespoon tamarind
concentrate (see Note)

4 cups warm water

25 drops liquid stevia,
or to taste

{ MAKES 4 CUPS }

Place the tamarind concentrate in a pitcher and pour in the 4 cups warm water. Stir to dissolve and add the stevia. Refrigerate until cold, and serve over ice.

NOTE: Tamarind is a sour-sweet tropical pod fruit widely used in Indian, Asian, African, and Latin American cooking, in both sweet and savory recipes. You can find tamarind concentrate, as well as blocks of compressed tamarind pods, in Mexican, Indian, and international grocery stores.

tomato ice water

4 large tomatoes, frozen (see Sidebar)

Sea salt

I never liked tomatoes as I was growing up. Even now, sometimes I want them, sometimes not. But tomato water—the clear liquid from the tomato—is another thing entirely. Tomato water was a trendy ingredient in upscale restaurants back in the 1980s. The object was to capture the pure essence of the fruit, slowly, by first pureeing the tomatoes, then stuffing them into cheesecloth, tying the cheesecloth to a wooden spoon, and suspending it overnight over a bowl to drain and release the tomato water.

My version bypasses all those time-consuming steps, and it can be made year-round because it uses frozen tomatoes. All you need to do is thaw the tomatoes. As they thaw, the clear liquid is released from the flesh, the skin peels right off, and, voilà, the water is ready for drinking or to be used as the base of any number of mixed drinks or soups.

Save the tomato flesh and use it as the base for my raw tomato Ketchup (page 105).

....

Place the tomatoes in a bowl and thaw them for 5 to 6 hours, until they release their clear liquid. Remove and discard the peel, place the tomatoes in a fine-mesh strainer, and squeeze until all the clear liquid comes out. Save the solids for another use and season the liquid with salt.

line them up and freeze them

When summer's nearing an end and you have a surplus of tomatoes in your garden or they are on sale in the supermarket, freeze a bunch of them. It's unlikely you'll get another good fresh tomato for a long time—winter tomatoes are often pale looking with little flavor. To freeze tomatoes, line some up on a baking sheet and freeze them solid. Then place them in freezer bags, seal the bags, and enjoy them throughout the cold-weather season.

watermelon agua fresca

{ **SERVES 1** }

4 cups seedless watermelon, cut into ½-inch cubes

½ cup water

Juice of 1 lime

2 tablespoons raw honey or raw agave nectar

This sweet and refreshing beverage can be found at roadside stands all over Mexico. Watermelon is mostly water, so enjoy yourself and don't worry that you're drinking too much sugar. Stir in a few mint leaves to add to the cooling effect.

Combine the ingredients in a blender with the ½ cup water and blend until smooth. Strain and serve over ice.

flavor tip

When serving your drinks on ice, to keep the flavor full strength, try freezing a portion of the beverage itself in ice cube trays and add the flavored ice cubes to your drinks. Or toss a few flavored ice cubes in sparkling water for just a hint of flavor.

TURN YOUR DRINK INTO DESSERT

You can transform any drink into a granita, an Italian-style frozen dessert (similar to Italian ices, but coarser), by simply freezing it. Pour your drink into a baking pan and freeze, scraping the pan every 30 minutes or so until almost completely frozen, about 3 hours. Then scrape the granita into bowls and serve. Tip: Freezing makes food taste less sweet, so you may want to increase the amount of sweetener before freezing.

chia fresca

{ SERVES 1 }

1¼ cups water

3 tablespoons fresh lime juice

2 tablespoons raw agave nectar or raw honey

1 tablespoon chia seeds

Chia seeds are amazingly versatile, and are good for my athlete boyfriend. Why? Because they absorb up to ten times their volume in water, which makes them amazingly hydrating. In fact, the Tarahumara tribe of Mexico, known as the world's first endurance runners, drink beverages made with chia seeds to sustain themselves on their typical hundred-mile runs. And before them the ancient Aztecs valued the seeds so much they used them as currency.

So pass on those store-bought energy drinks filled with shoddy ingredients and hydrate yourself with chia fresca. Or add a few seeds to your smoothies for an extra hit of fiber and some added thickness. See page 60 for more on chia seeds.

Pour the water into a tall glass. Add the lime juice and agave and whisk until the agave dissolves. Add the chia seeds, stir well to fully moisten them, and set aside for 10 minutes, stirring a couple of times to keep the seeds from sticking together.

timesaver
During active times, like training for a race, increase the recipe and have enough in your fridge to last you a week.

spreads, condiments, & dips

When you're having a party, try going raw. In my Turn It Raw chapter, I showed you how just about any recipe can go raw. Here you'll find raw versions of many of our typical pantry ingredients: nut butters, jams, ketchup, mustard, and pickles. You'll also find a selection of spreads, dips, salsa, guacamole, relish, and slaw recipes. Lots to choose from—so go ahead and spread, dip, and enjoy to your heart's content!

nutty butter

4 cups raw cashew pieces, soaked, and dried raw almonds (see Note), or other nuts

2 tablespoons cold-pressed extra-virgin olive oil

⅛ teaspoon sea salt

tip

It can be hard to scrape every last bit of nut butter from your blender, if that's what you used, so make your next smoothie in the blender and enjoy the leftover nut butter in your drink.

Freshly made nut butters are miles away in taste from those found in a jar, and they are very easy to make. For this job I prefer the food processor to my high-speed blender, as its wide blade easily reaches all the nuts and makes short work of them.

If you are using a food processor, place the nuts in the bowl of the processor and process until smooth, 8 to 10 minutes, scraping down the sides as needed and stopping the machine every couple of minutes so it doesn't get too hot. A couple of minutes before the nut butter is done, it will form a ball in the machine; continue to process until the oils from the nuts are released and the nut butter is smooth and creamy. Add the oil and salt and process briefly to combine.

If you are using a high-speed blender, place the nuts in the blender, cover, and blend on high speed (using the tamper if you're using a VitaMix) to work the nuts into a smooth nut butter, about 3 minutes, stopping the machine if it gets too hot.

Keep the nut butter in the refrigerator for up to 2 weeks.

NOTE: For almond butter, you will need to soak the almonds (see page 38) and dehydrate them for about 24 hours, until they are completely dry.

{ variations }

SWEET NUTTY BUTTER: Stir in 2 to 3 tablespoons raw honey or raw agave at the end.

CINNAMON-RAISIN NUTTY BUTTER: Stir in ½ teaspoon ground cinnamon and 2 tablespoons minced raisins at the end.

CHOCOLATE NUTTY BUTTER: Stir in ¼ cup raw cacao powder and 2 to 3 tablespoons raw honey or raw agave (the sweetener is optional) at the end.

NUTTY BUTTER WITH DRIED APPLES: Stir in 2 to 3 tablespoons minced dried apples at the end.

your fruit's in a jam

1 or 2 handfuls of dried fruit, such as prunes, dates, apples, or mangos, pitted if necessary

Raw honey, raw agave nectar, or coconut nectar to taste (optional)

tip
Add a touch of alcohol-free vanilla or almond extract, a little rosewater, or dried spices such as ground cinnamon, nutmeg, or cardamom. Experiment to come up with your own signature jam flavors!

Store-bought fruit jam is cooked and often filled with sugar or other sweeteners, and making it yourself is a time-consuming task. Though raw fruit jam made with dried fruit calls for overnight soaking, it can be put together in under five minutes of active time, and you decide how much sweetener it needs, depending on the sweetness of the fruit and personal preference.

When you buy dried fruits, make sure the label reads "sulfite free" (sulfur dioxide is a preservative that causes adverse reactions in some people) and "dehydrated." It should also be labeled "raw," as some dehydrated foods can be dried at temperatures higher than 115°F.

Place the dried fruit in a bowl and add water to cover. Set aside to soak overnight. Drain, reserving the soaking water, and place the fruit in a food processor. Process, adding reserved water as needed, until pureed. Taste and add some sweetener if needed. Store in the refrigerator for up to 2 weeks.

with pits or without?
Using pitted dates or prunes may save you a little time—it will take a few minutes to pit them yourself. But once the pits are removed, the fruit dries out more and loses some of its juiciness. Already pitted fruit is more difficult to process into a puree.

fig and rosemary jam

½ pound dried figs (about 2 cups), stems removed

¼ cup cold-pressed extra-virgin olive oil

2 tablespoons raw honey

1 teaspoon raw apple cider vinegar or coconut vinegar

Large pinch of sea salt

1 tablespoon minced fresh rosemary

This sweet-and-savory jam is wonderful spread over crackers (see pages 216 to 218 for recipes); top it with a slice of raw goat cheese to add a whole new dimension.

In a food processor or high-speed blender, combine all the ingredients except the rosemary. Add 3 tablespoons water, or as needed, and process until smooth. Add the rosemary and process briefly to combine. Store in a covered jar in the refrigerator for up to 2 weeks.

applesauce

4 medium apples, peeled, cored, and chopped

1 cup raisins

1 tablespoon fresh lemon juice

1 tablespoon chia seeds (optional)

Pinch of sea salt

We had an apple tree in our yard when I was growing up in New York. It's no longer there, but the memory of my mom's applesauce lives on—here in my raw take on her recipe. It's easy to fill up a bunch of minicontainers with this fresh-tasting applesauce and pack them in children's lunchboxes. Or spoon it over pancakes (see the recipes on pages 82 and 83) or cereal, or simply enjoy a bowl as a between-meal snack.

Combine all the ingredients in a food processor or high-speed blender and process for about 5 minutes, until very smooth.

{ variations }

CINNAMON APPLESAUCE: Add ¼ teaspoon ground cinnamon.

BERRY APPLESAUCE: Add ½ cup berries of your choice.

mayonnaise

1 large fertilized organic egg yolk (see page 50)

¼ teaspoon sea salt

2 teaspoons fresh lemon juice

½ cup raw neutral oil, such as cold-pressed sunflower oil (see Tips, below)

This is classic mayonnaise, so creamy and fresh tasting it's worth every turn of the whisk it takes to make. If you have concerns about raw eggs or are vegan, try the egg-free mayonnaise in the recipe on page 186. Add 3 to 4 tablespoons finely chopped Old World Cucumber Pickles (page 110) to turn this into tartar sauce.

In a medium bowl, combine the egg yolk and salt and whisk until well blended. Whisk in the lemon juice.

Drizzle in the oil, starting as slowly as you can, 1 or 2 drops at a time, whisking constantly. Once you've added about half of the oil, start adding the remaining oil in a very thin stream, whisking constantly. (You can also make it in a blender, adding the oil through the hole in the top in the same fashion as you blend.)

Place in a jar, cover, and store in the refrigerator for up to 4 days.

tips

- Put the oil in a squeeze bottle so you can add it slowly with ease.

- Keep all your ingredients at room temperature.

- Avoid using extra-virgin olive oil for mayonnaise, as its strong flavor dominates—but still use cold-pressed.

{ variations }

SPICY MAYONNAISE: Add ¼ teaspoon chipotle chile powder.

PESTO MAYONNAISE: Add 1 tablespoon pesto (pages 166 to 167).

HERB MAYONNAISE: Add ¼ cup minced fresh herbs, such as cilantro, basil, parsley, or mint, or a combination.

AIOLI: Add 1 garlic clove, pressed through a garlic press.

SAFFRON AIOLI: Add 1 garlic clove, pressed, and crumble in a large pinch of saffron.

the classics— mustard & ketchup

Eating raw foods is not about deprivation; it's about creativity and ingenuity and coming up with raw equivalents of cooked favorites, America's two favorite condiments—mustard and ketchup—included.

....

must-have mustard

{ MAKES ABOUT 1 CUP }

¼ cup yellow mustard seeds

¼ cup brown mustard seeds

½ cup raw apple cider vinegar

1 tablespoon raw honey or raw agave nectar

½ teaspoon sea salt

In a medium bowl, combine both mustard seeds with the vinegar. Add ½ cup water, stir, and cover loosely. Place on the counter for about 12 hours or overnight.

Place the soaked mixture in a high-speed blender, add the honey and salt, and blend until creamy, adding more water if needed. Refrigerate for 2 to 3 days before using to allow the flavors to settle and to mellow the bite of the mustard (it will be surprisingly sharp at first!). It will keep for about 2 weeks, covered, in the refrigerator.

ketchup

{ MAKES ABOUT ⅔ CUP }

4 tomatoes, frozen (see page 95)

2 tablespoons raw honey or raw agave nectar, or to taste (depending on how sweet the tomatoes are)

2 teaspoons raw apple cider vinegar

½ teaspoon tomato concentrate (optional; see Sources, page 239)

⅛ teaspoon ground turmeric

⅛ teaspoon ground ginger

¼ teaspoon sea salt, or to taste

Place the tomatoes in a bowl and let them thaw for 5 to 6 hours, until they release their liquid. Peel the tomatoes, put them in a fine-mesh strainer, and squeeze over a bowl until all the liquid is out.

Combine the tomato solids with the remaining ingredients in a blender or food processor and process until smooth. Strain through a coarse-mesh strainer to remove the seeds, pressing down to extract all the paste. Place in a jar, cover, and refrigerate until ready to use. The ketchup will keep for about 1 week.

sesame salt

½ cup raw unhulled sesame seeds

1 tablespoon sea salt

This is a delicious way to take advantage of the nutritional value and nutty flavor of sesame seeds while salting your food. It is based on a condiment called gomasio, a roasted sesame salt that is used widely in macrobiotic food. This version skips the roasting. Sprinkle it over vegetable and grain dishes anywhere you would normally use plain salt to add some depth of flavor and crunch.

The traditional vessel used to make sesame salt is called a suribachi, a bowl with a ridged pattern to facilitate grinding and a pestle made from wood to keep the ridges from wearing down. But any mortar and pestle or a quick pulse in a coffee grinder will do just fine.

The traditional ratio is 8 to 1 sesame seeds to salt, so you can scale the recipe up or down as you like. You can keep the sesame seeds whole as well, but grinding them makes their nutrients more absorbable. And nutrients they have aplenty: They are loaded with the minerals manganese and copper, and they are also a good source of calcium, magnesium, iron, phosphorus, zinc, and fiber.

Combine the sesame seeds and salt in a mortar and grind with a pestle until most of the seeds are cracked open, using just enough pressure to crack the seeds so their oil is released and coats each grain of salt. Alternatively, pulse in a coffee grinder, taking care not to grind too much or the seeds will turn into flour; you want to keep the texture of the seeds.

{ variations }

GARLIC SESAME SALT: Add ½ teaspoon garlic powder.

ONION SESAME SALT: Add ½ teaspoon onion powder.

DULSE SESAME SALT: Add 1 tablespoon dulse flakes.

pico de gallo

4 medium tomatoes, seeded and chopped

½ red onion, diced

1 garlic clove, minced

1 jalapeño chile, minced

½ cup chopped fresh cilantro

Juice of 1 lime

½ teaspoon sea salt

½ teaspoon chili powder

Pico de gallo, also called salsa fresca, is a fresh salsa prepared with less liquid than a typical salsa, making it a good choice for spooning over sandwiches and the like without getting your food soggy. Try it on an Ezekiel corn tortilla (see Sources, page 239) with avocado, shredded raw cheese, and a little lettuce or as a standard table condiment for a Mexican meal.

Place all of the ingredients in a large bowl, and stir well to combine. Store in a covered container in the refrigerator for up to 3 days.

{ variations }

MANGO PICO DE GALLO: Add 1 firm-ripe mango, peeled, pitted, and diced.

CUCUMBER PICO DE GALLO: Add 1 small cucumber, seeded and diced.

ginger-chile pickled carrots

{ **MAKES ABOUT 1 QUART** }

4 cups tightly packed grated carrots

2 tablespoons peeled, grated fresh ginger

2 heads garlic, peeled and grated or finely chopped

2 small chiles, finely chopped

2 tablespoons sea salt

Perched atop a mountain in Halifax, Vermont, Leah Mutz's Annamari Farm has a short growing season, so Leah grows an abundance of vegetables that she pickles and delivers to local clients throughout the long winter months. For those of us (me included!) who are more likely to pick their carrots from a supermarket shelf than out of the ground, Leah has shared her simple recipe here, so you can pickle them at home. All the ingredients—and the mason jars—can be found in your local grocery store.

This recipe is a perfect starter pickle for people who think they don't like fermented foods, as the sweetness of the carrots offsets the sour pickled taste, while the hits of garlic and spice give it a wonderful punch. (Feel free to add more ginger, garlic, and/or chiles to bump it up a few notches.) And unlike cucumber pickles, these carrots don't need a brine. So satisfying, it's like a summer salad preserved all through the winter! In fact, you can serve it in place of regular salad in the cold-weather months, or alongside any dinner entree.

While these carrots aren't difficult to make, they do require some patience—it will take 3 days to 2 weeks until they are ready to eat.

Combine all the ingredients in a large nonreactive bowl and pound with a meat mallet to thoroughly masticate the mixture, squeezing it with your hands to release the juices.

Place the mixture in a clean half-gallon, wide-mouth glass jar or small crock and press down firmly until the carrots are packed tight and the brine covers the carrots. If after pressing down on the carrots you can't seem to get the brine to climb over the surface of the carrots, make a brine of 1 tablespoon sea salt for every 1 cup water, and go ahead and add as much of it as you need to get the carrots covered in liquid.

Weight the carrots down with a jar filled with water (or another heavy object that fits inside the mouth of your original jar), and press down on the weight. Finally, cover the whole works with a clean dishtowel. Push down on the weight as often as you think of it, at least once a day. Scrape away any mold that forms on the surface of the brine, but don't worry if you can't get it all. Now don't get put off by the word "mold." The level of salt in the pickle makes it uninhabitable for any harmful bacteria. The bad stuff just can't grow while saturated in that level of salt. Mold grows on the top because it is exposed to the air, so if you scrape off as much mold as you can and stir in the few particles that are left, there is nothing to worry about.

Leave for 3 days. Then taste the carrots every day, and when they are tangy and fermented enough to your liking, between 3 days and 2 weeks, transfer the carrots and brine to a clean quart-size mason jar. Pack them tightly, cover, and refrigerate. They will keep for about a year.

old world cucumber pickles

Enough cucumbers to loosely fill a 1-gallon glass crock or jar (about 2 dozen small cucumbers)

¼ cup plus 2 tablespoons sea salt

2 quarts pure water (see Notes)

3 to 4 heads fresh flowering dill, or 3 to 4 tablespoons dried dill or dill seeds

2 to 3 heads garlic, peeled

10 black peppercorns

5 to 7 fresh grape leaves (optional; see Notes)

I loved pickles so much as a kid that I would take a spoon and eat the seeds out of them and then savor the skin last—so I consider myself a pickle expert of sorts!

What makes these pickles different from the ones you buy on the shelf? First and foremost, taste: They have a sour flavor with a hint of effervescence, and the dill and garlic are subtle enough that they don't knock you over the head with every bite. Second, crispness: Traditional pickles retain their crunch in a way that other pickles don't. Third, health: They are totally raw and chock-full of healthy bacteria and nutrients that will nourish your body. Small to medium fresh firm cucumbers, or pickling cucumbers, generally are preferred, as they hold up best in the brine. What to make your pickles in? Ceramic crocks are ideal, though a little pricey. You can also use a 1-gallon plastic bucket, as long as it is food-grade plastic. Often supermarket delis will give these away if you ask. Do not use metal.

This recipe also comes from Leah Mutz of Annamari Farm, in Vermont. Leah explains that her recipe follows the age-old Eastern European tradition of naturally fermenting cucumbers into sour pickles. Most of the pickles you find at the supermarket nowadays are cured in vinegar, which reduces their nutritional level by destroying their enzymes. But when you ferment your pickles naturally, you end up with more nutrients than when you started, making them cucumbers plus! Note that it will take 1 to 4 weeks for the cucumbers to turn into pickles.

Gently rinse the cucumbers, taking care not to bruise them.

In a large pitcher or a bowl, stir the salt into the water until it is completely dissolved. Combine the dill, garlic, peppercorns, and grape leaves, if using, in the bottom of a clean 1-gallon crock, and then place the clean cucumbers on top. Pour the salt brine over the cucumbers.

Find a plate that fits snugly inside the crock and place it on the cucumbers. Now find a weight that fits in the crock as well (a clean gallon mason jar works well) and place it on the plate. Press down until the brine rises over the level of the plate. If you need more brine to cover the plate, mix a solution of 1 tablespoon salt for every 1 cup water and add as much as you need.

Cover the mouth of the crock with a clean cloth and check your pickles every day until they are soured to your liking; this will take 1 to 4 weeks. In the meantime, scrape away any mold that forms on the surface of the brine, but don't worry if you can't get it all (see page 109, where I address the issue of mold). If the plate and weight become moldy, rinse them before replacing them. Transfer the pickles and brine to clean mason jars, cover, and refrigerate. They will keep for about a year.

NOTES: Use only pure water—spring water, filtered water, or well water—nothing that has a chlorine smell to it. Chlorine inhibits the growth of microbes, and we need some of those good guys to make the fermentation happen.

Tannin-rich grape leaves are the secret to the crunchiest pickles, so it's worth looking around for a neighbor with a grapevine.

pineapple salsa

1 cup finely chopped fresh pineapple

1 green bell pepper, cored, seeded, and diced

1 cup fresh corn kernels (see opposite)

1 small red onion, finely chopped

½ cup sprouted black beans (see page 39; optional)

1 jalapeño chile, seeded and minced

2 tablespoons fresh lime juice

½ teaspoon ground cumin

½ teaspoon sea salt

¼ cup chopped fresh cilantro

I'm not a person who likes to mix fruit and "real" food—to me fruit has its place separate from meals. Here I make an exception. And eating the colors of the rainbow comes easily with this salsa: yellow pineapple and corn, green pepper, red onion, and black beans—you've got them all. Try serving it with seared fish or in tiny bowls all on its own. You can also try substituting mango for the pineapple.

In a large bowl, combine all the ingredients and stir well. Store in a covered container in the refrigerator for up to 3 days.

NO NEED TO GAS UP!

If you're new to sprouting, you may need a little help digesting sprouted beans. Try this Indian digestion secret: Chew on a few ajwain seeds. Ajwain seeds taste like a cross between thyme and caraway. They counter the gassy effects of beans and are good for digestion in general. They can be found in any Indian grocery store.

timesaver

You only need 1 cup of pineapple, so save yourself the fuss of peeling and chopping and buy a small container of fresh pineapple chunks in the produce section of your supermarket.

corn relish

1 cup corn kernels

2 tablespoons fresh lime juice

½ teaspoon plus a pinch of sea salt

½ medium red onion, finely chopped

½ green bell pepper, cored, seeded, and finely chopped

1 small cucumber, finely chopped

1 garlic clove, pressed through a garlic press

Serve this tangy relish alongside sandwiches or seared fish or meat, or spoon some over a bowl of soup for added texture. To turn the relish into a salad, add 1 cup halved cherry tomatoes; serve over a sprouted grain (page 39), and you have lunch. For the real taste of summer, make this relish in season with fresh rather than frozen corn kernels.

In a medium bowl, combine the corn, lime juice, and a pinch of salt. Set aside to marinate for 1 hour. Add the remaining ½ teaspoon salt, onion, bell pepper, cucumber, and garlic. Store in a covered container in the refrigerator for up to 3 days.

BUNDT PANS AREN'T JUST FOR BAKING

Trying to cut kernels off the cob can be trying, as it's a challenge to keep those kernels from flying off the cutting board and all over the kitchen floor. The solution: Repurpose your Bundt pan (that tall, round cake pan with a hole in the middle) as a corn stand. (A tube pan will do the job as well.)

Shuck your ear of corn, then position it, tip end down, in the hole in the middle of the pan and hold onto the stem end. Run a sharp knife down the ear, shaving off the kernels. Rotate the ear to remove the kernels from all sides; they will drop tidily into the bottom of the pan, ready to be put to use. If you don't have a Bundt pan, a large, wide bowl will do the trick: Set the tip of your ear of corn at the bottom of the bowl on an angle and shave off the kernels, rotating the ear as you would for the Bundt pan method.

jícama slaw

1 medium jícama,
coarsely grated

1 medium carrot,
coarsely grated

½ cup Mayonnaise
(page 104)

2 tablespoons fresh
lime juice

1 tablespoon raw honey
or raw agave nectar
(optional)

½ teaspoon ground
cumin

¼ teaspoon sea salt,
or to taste

¼ teaspoon freshly
ground black pepper

Pinch of cayenne
pepper

¼ cup chopped fresh
cilantro, basil, or mint

This slaw recipe uses crunchy and slightly sweet jícama rather than the standard cabbage. Any crisp root vegetable can make a great slaw—roots that you normally wouldn't think of, such as daikon, turnips, celeriac, or kohlrabi. Feel free to experiment with your favorites.

Combine the jícama and carrot in a large bowl.

In a small bowl, whisk together the mayonnaise, lime juice, honey, if using, cumin, salt, black pepper, and cayenne. Add to the jícama and toss to coat. Stir in the cilantro. Store in a covered container in the refrigerator for up to 3 days.

{ variation }

JÍCAMA APPLE SLAW: Add 1 green apple, peeled, cored, and shredded.

tomatillo guacamole

{ **MAKES ABOUT 3 CUPS** }

1 garlic clove

½ jalapeño chile
(seeded if you like
your guacamole mild)

½ pound tomatillos,
husked and washed

½ teaspoon sea salt

2 large ripe avocados

½ small red onion,
finely chopped

½ cup chopped fresh
cilantro

tip
To prevent your
guacamole from turning
brown, press plastic
wrap directly onto the
surface, so the plastic
touches it and keeps
the air out. Store in a
covered container in
the refrigerator for
up to 3 days.

The tomatillo—a member of the tomato family—is a small fruit a
little larger than the cherry tomato but green in color and covered
with a papery husk that you remove before using. It is tangy, so this
guacamole doesn't need lime like traditional guacamole. Serve with
crackers or crudités, or alongside a salad.

Turn on the food processor and drop the garlic clove through
the feed tube. Then drop the jalapeño in. Turn off the machine
and add the tomatillos and salt. Process until pureed, with small
pieces remaining.

Cut the avocados in half, remove their pits, and scoop their
flesh into a bowl. Mash the avocados coarsely with a fork or
potato masher. Add the onion, then add the pureed tomatillos,
and stir to combine. Stir in the cilantro.

plantain guacamole

1 very ripe plantain, halved crosswise and middle string removed

2 ripe medium avocados, halved, pitted, and flesh scooped out

1 small red onion, finely chopped

3 tablespoons fresh lime juice

1 jalapeño chile (seeded if you like your guacamole mild)

½ teaspoon sea salt

½ cup chopped fresh cilantro

I'm a guac girl—and here is a different take on guacamole, with plantains adding a sweet twist. Make sure your plantains are very ripe before using them: Once they are completely black, soft, and sweet, rather than starchy, they are perfect for eating in the raw. Serve with crackers or crudités.

Scoop the plantain from its skin with a spoon; use a grapefruit spoon if you have one.

In a large bowl, combine all the ingredients except the cilantro and mash with a fork or potato masher until fairly smooth, with some visible chunks remaining. Or use a mortar and pestle. Stir in the cilantro and serve immediately.

creamy red pepper dip

{ **MAKES ABOUT 1 CUP** }

1 small red bell pepper, cored, seeded, and chopped

1 cup raw cashews, soaked (see page 38)

¼ cup chopped raw green olives

2 tablespoons cold-pressed olive oil

2 tablespoons unpasteurized white miso

¼ teaspoon ground turmeric

Pinch of cayenne pepper

1 teaspoon raw apple cider vinegar

½ teaspoon onion powder

1 teaspoon minced fresh chives or other herb (optional)

The cashew, so versatile and mild in taste, makes a great base for a host of raw recipes: ice cream, cereals, and cream, to name a few. Here it adds creaminess to this luscious dip, which can be used in place of cheese or dairy dips. The red pepper—along with a little turmeric—provides a hint of sweetness and a vibrant orange color.

In a high-speed blender or food processor, combine all the ingredients except the chives and blend until smooth, using the blender's tamper or scraping the sides of the food processor as needed. Stir in the chives. Cover and refrigerate for up to 1 week.

okima's nori cheese

{ MAKES 4 ROLLS }

1 cup raw cashews, soaked, with their soaking water (see page 38; soak in about 1½ cups water)

¼ cup fresh lemon juice

2 tablespoons nutritional yeast

1 tablespoon kelp or dulse flakes

1 garlic clove

1 teaspoon sea salt

4 sheets raw nori

Basic Flax Crackers (page 216), for serving

I was the keynote speaker at the Navel Expo on wellness on Long Island when I first met Okima Wilcox-Hitt of Live Island Cafe (www.liveislandcafe.com) in Huntington, New York, Long Island's first and only all-raw eatery. Thank you, Okima, for bringing raw closer to my family on Long Island. This clever vegan cheese recipe makes a wonderful addition to a raw cheese platter—great for entertaining. If you'd like a firmer cheese, you can dehydrate the rolls at 115°F for 12 to 24 hours.

In a high-speed blender or food processor, blend the cashews with their soaking water until a thick cream is formed. Add the lemon juice, nutritional yeast, kelp, garlic, and salt and blend until smooth. Transfer to a bowl, cover, and refrigerate the cheese until fairly firm, about 2 hours.

Lay out a sheet of nori and spread ¼ cup of the chilled cheese over the bottom half of the nori sheet. Roll up sushi style, and repeat with the remaining nori and cheese. Refrigerate until ready to serve. To serve, slice the roll and serve with flax crackers. The uncut nori rolls will keep, covered and refrigerated, for 3 to 5 days.

room for 'shrooms and walnut pâté

{ MAKES ABOUT 2 CUPS }

1 pound white
mushrooms, chopped

½ cup cold-pressed
extra-virgin olive oil

2 tablespoons raw
apple cider vinegar,
or to taste

3 garlic cloves, pressed
through a garlic press

½ teaspoon dried sage

½ teaspoon dried
thyme

¼ teaspoon sea salt,
or to taste

¼ teaspoon freshly
ground black pepper

1 cup raw walnuts,
soaked (see page 38)

1 tablespoon nutritional
yeast

1 tablespoon fresh
lemon juice, or to taste

Mushroom lovers, this dish is for you! As dehydrating concentrates flavor, the end result is a pâté with a heightened earthy mushroom flavor. The walnuts give it body and creaminess, and the herbs and spices bring it all together. Spread it over crackers or bread, or use it as a dip for vegetables.

In a large bowl, combine the mushrooms, oil, vinegar, garlic, sage, thyme, salt, and pepper and toss to coat the mushrooms well. Spread out on a ParaFlexx-lined dehydrator tray and place in the dehydrator. Set the machine to 105°F and dehydrate for 1½ to 2 hours, until the mushrooms are soft.

Transfer the mushrooms to a food processor, scraping the seasoned oil from the ParaFlexx sheet, and add the walnuts, nutritional yeast, and lemon juice. Process until smooth, 2 to 3 minutes, scraping down the sides of the machine a few times. Taste and add more vinegar, lemon juice, and/or salt if needed. Cover and refrigerate for up to 1 week.

{ variation }

MARINATED MUSHROOMS: Follow the above steps through dehydrating the mushrooms and you're done. (Omit the walnuts, yeast, and lemon juice.) They taste just like roasted mushrooms and can be eaten as a vegetable side or in a salad.

the goddess is green dip

1 ripe avocado, halved, pitted, and flesh scooped out

½ cup Mayonnaise (page 104)

1 shallot, chopped

1 garlic clove

1 tablespoon fresh lemon juice, or to taste

⅛ teaspoon sea salt, or to taste

¼ teaspoon freshly ground black pepper

2 scallions, white and green parts, finely chopped

1 tablespoon minced fresh herbs, such as chives, parsley, or dill, or a combination; or 1 teaspoon dried herbs

2 teaspoons dulse flakes (optional)

This version of the classic green goddess dressing gets its color from avocados rather than pureed herbs, and dulse flakes take the place of the standard anchovies. Trivia fact: Green goddess dressing is named not for its color, but for a play called *The Green Goddess*. The dressing was created for an event in the 1920s celebrating the production.

In a food processor or blender, combine the avocado, mayonnaise, 2 tablespoons water, the shallot, garlic, lemon juice, salt, and pepper and process until smooth.

Transfer to a bowl and stir in the scallions, herbs, and dulse flakes, if using. Taste and add more lemon juice and/or salt if needed and more water if it is too thick. Cover and refrigerate for up to 2 days.

{ variation }

GREEN GODDESS SPREAD: To turn the dip into a super-creamy spread, omit the water.

salads & salad dressings

Salads truly are the most fun you can have with food—just add whatever vegetables you like. And you can get a salad anywhere. What you cannot get just anywhere is a fabulous raw salad dressing. So this is where I will help you to excel.

When you go raw, salads will naturally become a large part of your world; they will become your go-to dish or your plan B if you find yourself in that rare species of restaurant that has absolutely no raw food, or at least no raw food that you trust to be safe. Read on to see how simple it is to make your own dressings. Man, they will jazz up any bowl of greens—you'll never be bored by salad again. You may even choose to eat salads every day!

essential herb vinaigrette

¼ cup raw apple cider vinegar or coconut vinegar

½ cup cold-pressed extra-virgin olive oil

1 tablespoon fresh lemon or lime juice

1 tablespoon raw honey or raw agave nectar

½ teaspoon onion powder (optional)

½ teaspoon garlic powder (optional)

½ teaspoon sea salt

1 tablespoon minced fresh herbs, such as oregano, rosemary, or basil, or a combination; or 1 teaspoon dried herbs

I wish I had had this dressing when my dad made grilled steak, his specialty. I was not a meat lover and doused my steak (to his dismay) with Caesar dressing from a bottle!

The key to making a first-rate salad dressing is getting the proportions right: the correct amount of vinegar or citrus to give it some zing, a little sweetener to balance it out, and enough salt to pull it all together. Good-quality salt doesn't just make your food taste salty. In addition to being chock-full of minerals and other nutrients (see page 55), it makes other ingredients taste better because it brings out their natural flavors.

In a blender, combine all the ingredients except the herbs and blend until emulsified. Add the herbs and pulse to combine. Alternatively, combine all the ingredients in a jar, cover with the lid, and shake until the mixture is emulsified.

herbs: fresh and dried

The flavor of dried herbs is more concentrated than that of fresh herbs. The rule of thumb is to use a third less dried herbs than you would fresh, and likewise, three times as much fresh herbs as dried.

my on-the-go dressing starter

2 parts cold-pressed extra-virgin olive oil

1 part Udo's Choice Oil Blend (see page 58)

Sea salt

I never leave home without packing a little vial of raw dressing starter. I order my salad undressed with a lemon on the side, then I discreetly pour on a little starter from my secret stash. Here is my quick and easy formula.

In a little vial, combine the two oils. Order a salad with lemon wedges on the side, shake the dressing, and pour. Squeeze the lemon over the salad and sprinkle with salt.

IS THAT SALAD DRESSING IN YOUR PURSE, OR ARE YOU JUST GLAD TO SEE ME?

Guilty as charged. If I'm going to cheat, I'm not going to waste it on cooked oil in my supposedly slimming salad (I'll take the popcorn, thank you very much). Most restaurant salads are made with cooked dressing: even extra-virgin olive oil isn't raw unless it's cold-pressed. I prefer to avoid grilling the waitstaff to figure out which oil they use (because they never know) and bring my own.

easiest umeboshi vinaigrette

¾ cup cold-pressed extra-virgin olive oil or Udo's Choice Oil Blend (see page 58)

1 tablespoon umeboshi vinegar

Umeboshi is a Japanese plum that's dried and naturally pickled. With a delicate pink color and a sour, tart, and fruity flavor, umeboshi vinegar is used as an ingredient in dressings and sauces and is sprinkled over vegetables in any number of dishes. Try it in my Kale and Avocado Salad (page 137) or any salad of your choosing.

Technically speaking, umeboshi vinegar is not a vinegar because it contains salt. When you're making dressing, that means one less step—just add your oil and you're good to go. The umeboshi plum is a tiny thumb-size fruit that is traditionally dried and served as a condiment; it adds a burst of flavor to any dish. You can find umeboshi vinegar at natural foods stores.

In a small bowl, combine the oil and vinegar and whisk until emulsified. Alternatively, combine the ingredients in a jar with a lid, cover, and shake until emulsified. Whisk or shake again just before dressing your salad. Store in a covered container in the refrigerator for up to 2 weeks.

spice is nice cumin and garlic dressing

{ **MAKES ABOUT ½ CUP** }

Juice of 2 limes

1 jalapeño chile, minced

2 garlic cloves, minced

¼ teaspoon sea salt

¼ teaspoon freshly ground black pepper

¼ cup cold-pressed extra-virgin olive oil

1 teaspoon cumin seeds

Add a little heat to your salads with this Mexican-inspired dressing. Try tossing it with a mix of watercress, scallions, and shredded carrots or a simple arugula salad.

In a small bowl, combine the lime juice, jalapeño, garlic, salt, and pepper. Slowly whisk in the oil and add the cumin seeds. Alternatively, combine all the ingredients in a jar with a lid, cover, and shake until emulsified. Store in a covered container in the refrigerator for up to 3 days.

WHITE-HOT HEAT

To tame the heat of chiles, don't just remove the seeds. Remove the white membranes surrounding the seeds, too, as they are the hottest part of the chile.

raspberry vinaigrette

{ **MAKES 1 CUP** }

1 pint raspberries

1 tablespoon raw apple cider vinegar

1 tablespoon raw honey or raw agave nectar

¼ cup cold-pressed olive oil or Udo's Choice Oil Blend (see page 58)

1 tablespoon minced fresh mint

Sea salt and freshly ground black pepper

Fruity, sweet, tart, and bursting with antioxidants and vitamins—what more could you ask for in a dressing?

Place the raspberries in a food processor and puree until smooth. Strain through a fine-mesh strainer into a bowl, pressing on the solids to extract all the juice. Discard the seeds.

Whisk the vinegar and honey into the juice, then slowly whisk in the oil until emulsified. Add the mint and season with salt and pepper. Store in a covered container in the refrigerator for up to 2 days.

tip

Make the vinaigrette with frozen berries (thaw them first). You'll be blending them up anyway, so no one will know the difference!

blue cheese vinaigrette

{ **MAKES ABOUT 1 CUP** }

¾ cup cold-pressed olive oil or Udo's Choice Oil Blend (page 58)

2 tablespoons raw apple cider vinegar

1 tablespoon Must-Have Mustard (page 105) or prepared raw mustard

1 garlic clove

¼ teaspoon sea salt

A few grinds of black pepper

1 cup crumbled raw blue cheese

tip
Pair blue cheese with anything fruity or sweet for a great flavor contrast.

Serve this sophisticated take on blue cheese dressing with romaine wedges, apples, and walnuts, as a dip for crudité, or drizzled over a lightly seared steak (page 70).

In a blender, combine all the ingredients except 2 tablespoons of the cheese. Blend until emulsified. Stir in the reserved crumbled cheese. Store in a covered container in the refrigerator for up to 2 days.

CHOOSING RAW-MILK CHEESES
Go to your supermarket, Whole Foods, or international cheese store and ask to taste their raw-milk cheeses. They should have a variety of cheeses: hard and soft, from the milk of cows, goats, and sheep. Try them all and decide which ones you like.

timesaver
Buy a package of blue cheese crumbles—just make sure they are raw (Trader Joe's carries them).

carrot-ginger dressing

3 medium carrots, chopped

One 2-inch piece fresh ginger, peeled and chopped

⅓ cup water, or as needed

¼ cup raw apple cider vinegar

2 shallots, chopped

1 garlic clove

1 tablespoon nama shoyu

1 tablespoon raw honey or raw agave nectar

1 teaspoon unpasteurized sweet white miso

¾ cup cold-pressed sesame oil, cold-pressed extra-virgin olive oil, or Udo's Choice Oil Blend (see page 58)

This is my all-time favorite dressing, my version of the ever-popular bright orange dressing served over salad in Japanese restaurants, and it's better because I know it's raw. I sometimes have it on the side with my sashimi for something a little different.

In a high-speed blender, combine the carrots, ginger, water, and vinegar and blend until smooth, adding a little more water if needed to fully blend the ingredients. Add the remaining ingredients and blend until smooth, adding more water or oil to thin out the dressing if needed. Store in a covered container in the refrigerator for up to 3 days.

mango lassi, PAGE 92

light as a feather
apple chips, PAGE 230

good stuff by mom & me's salad pizza with mama claire's pesto sauce, PAGE 178

good stuff by mom & me's salad pizza with tomato sauce, PAGE 175

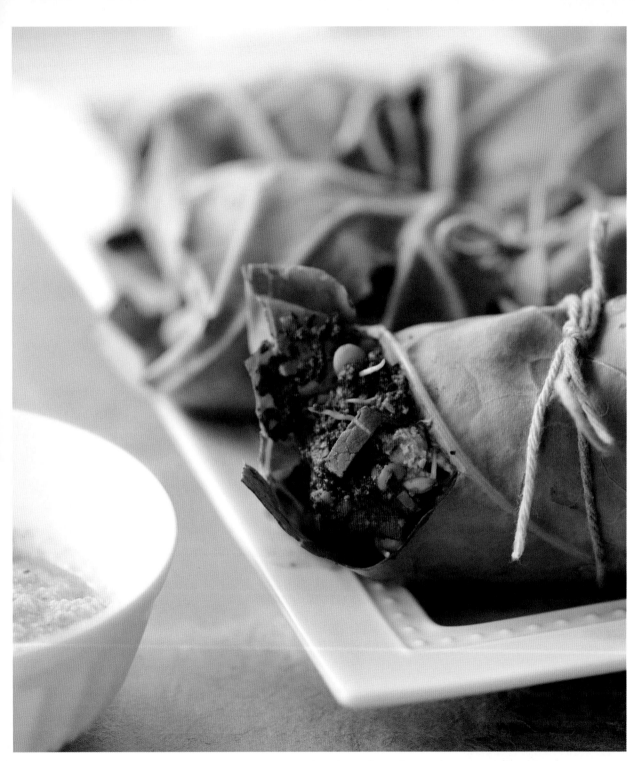

beet and cashew cheese collard tacos, PAGE 170

prune and chia porridge, PAGE 79

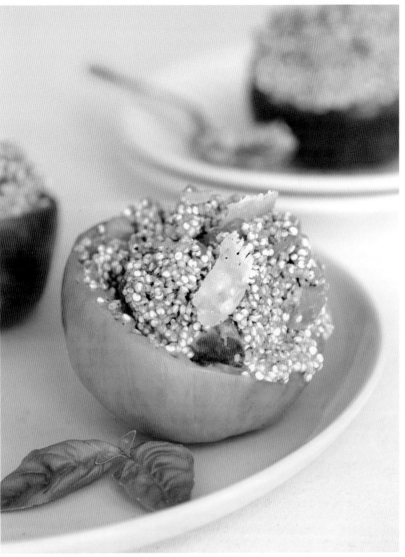

quinoa and
pesto–stuffed
tomatoes, PAGE 152

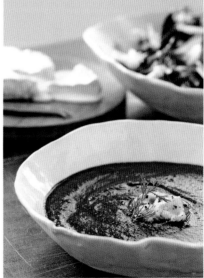

fennel and
radicchio salad
with raspberry
vinaigrette, PAGE 135

tangy live
borscht, PAGE 148

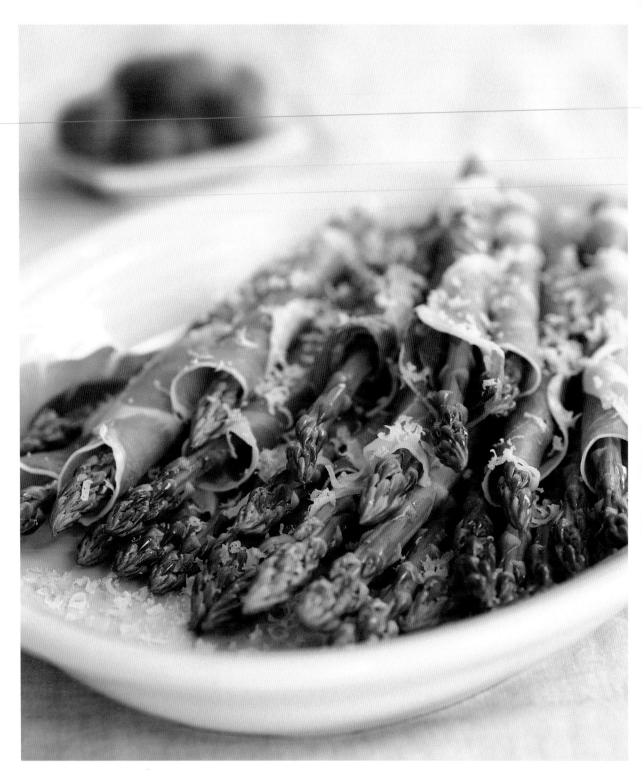

prosciutto-wrapped
asparagus spears,
PAGE 151

kelp noodles with
tahini sauce, PAGE 165

frozen chocolate
truffles, PAGE 197

maya
chocolate
pie, PAGE 203

honey mustard seed vinaigrette

{ **MAKES ABOUT 1½ CUPS** }

⅓ cup raw honey

2 tablespoons Must-Have Mustard (page 105) or prepared raw mustard

1 tablespoon fresh lemon juice

¼ cup raw apple cider vinegar

1 shallot, quartered

1 garlic clove

1 cup cold-pressed extra-virgin olive oil or Udo's Choice Oil Blend (see page 58)

Pinch of sea salt

2 teaspoons yellow mustard seeds

2 teaspoons brown mustard seeds

This dressing is sweet, tangy, and creamy even without the mayo that's usually added to dressings like this, and the mustard seeds give it a nice little bite and some texture. It's great over any salad, or try tossing with zucchini noodles (see page 166) or drizzling over flatbread (pages 220 and 221) in a prosciutto and raw cheese sandwich.

In a blender, combine the honey, mustard, lemon juice, vinegar, shallot, and garlic and process until smooth. With the motor on, gradually add the oil in a steady stream through the hole in the lid until smooth and creamy. Transfer to a bowl or jar and stir in the salt and mustard seeds. Store in a covered container in the refrigerator for up to 3 days.

when the pickings are slim

When you're eating out and you can't find anything raw on the menu, don't be shy about requesting a special-order salad with any and every vegetable they have in the kitchen. Just tell them not to cook those vegetables! Any chef worth her salt is up for a good challenge, and your salad might wind up being the best dish on the table.

nothing to sneeze at creamy black pepper and herb dressing

{ **MAKES ABOUT 2 CUPS** }

¾ cup raw sesame tahini

2 tablespoons unpasteurized sweet white miso

½ teaspoon sea salt

½ cup cold-pressed extra-virgin olive oil or Udo's Choice Oil Blend (see page 58)

1 tablespoon freshly ground black pepper

2 tablespoons fresh lemon juice

2 tablespoons raw honey or raw agave nectar

½ cup water, or more as needed

½ cup chopped fresh herbs, such as tarragon, sage, parsley, or dill

Even though I'm not vegan, I appreciate the many ways to make a dressing creamy without the cream, and using tahini is one of my favorites. This dressing continues to thicken as it sits; add water to thin it out as needed.

In a food processor, combine all the ingredients except the herbs and process until smooth, adding more water if needed. Add the herbs and pulse until minced. Store in a covered container in the refrigerator for up to 3 days.

down on the ranch dressing

{ **MAKES ABOUT 1½ CUPS** }

1 cup thick Basic Kefir
(page 90)

1 cup raw macadamia
nuts, soaked in water to
cover for 1 hour

1 or 2 Medjool dates,
pitted and halved

2 teaspoons raw apple
cider vinegar

2 tablespoons fresh
lemon juice

2 teaspoons garlic
powder

2 teaspoons onion
powder

1 teaspoon sea salt

¼ teaspoon freshly
ground black pepper

1 tablespoon finely
chopped fresh parsley

1 tablespoon finely
chopped fresh chives

The secret to the ranch taste is using garlic and onion powder—in this case, believe it or not, fresh isn't necessarily best! Depending on how thick your kefir is, you may need to add a little water to thin the dressing out—or keep the mixture thick and use it as a dip. If the kefir is particularly tangy, you may want to add the second date to sweeten it up.

In a high-speed blender, combine the kefir, macadamias, date, vinegar, lemon juice, garlic powder, onion powder, salt, and pepper and blend until smooth and creamy. Add the parsley and chives and pulse to combine. Store in a covered container in the refrigerator for up to 3 days.

{ variation }
If you don't have kefir on hand but you do have raw dairy milk, make a quick buttermilk: Add 1 tablespoon fresh lemon juice to 1 cup raw milk and let stand for 10 minutes; use in place of the kefir.

basil chia seed dressing

2 tablespoons chia
seeds

¾ cup water

1 tablespoon fresh lime
or lemon juice

1 tablespoon raw
apple cider vinegar
or coconut vinegar

2 teaspoons raw honey
or agave nectar

½ teaspoon sea salt

Pinch of freshly ground
black pepper

¾ cup cold-pressed
extra-virgin olive oil

¾ cup chopped fresh
basil

Chia seeds have amazing thickening powers—we've turned them into porridge (page 79), we've used them to add bulk to an energy drink (page 76), and here we blend them into a salad dressing that's so thick and creamy it's hard to believe it's dairy free. Note that the chia seeds need to be soaked for at least 6 hours, so plan ahead.

In a small bowl, combine the chia seeds and water and leave to soak for about 6 hours or overnight to dissolve the chia seeds; they will turn into a gel.

In a blender, combine the chia gel, lime juice, vinegar, honey, salt, and pepper and blend until smooth. With the motor running, pour the oil through the hole in the lid in a slow, steady stream to emulsify the dressing. Add the basil and blend until smooth and a vibrant green color. Store in a covered container in the refrigerator for up to 3 days.

{ variation }

Substitute a combination of mint and cilantro for the basil.

empty the fridge salad

Anybody can make a salad, but can they make a great salad? It's a heck of a lot easier to use up what's in your fridge than to shop for six or seven different vegetables and follow a recipe, so think of this more as a guideline to take what you've got and make it really flavorful, rather than a carved-in-stone recipe. This is the salad I fix—in one form or another—just about every day, switching it up here and there to keep things interesting.

1. Fill a salad bowl with some greens—arugula, red leaf, Boston, whatever looks good.

2. Toss it with some Udo's Choice Oil Blend (see page 58) and cold-pressed extra-virgin olive oil and perhaps a squeeze of lemon juice.

3. Add a little raw nama shoyu, nutritional flakes, and sea salt.

4. Crack an egg right into the bowl and toss it in (yep, a whole egg, but always a fertilized one; see page 51); if you are vegan or have concerns about raw eggs, skip it.

5. Choose your toppings: a raw cheese such as Emmenthaler, avocado, sunflower or other seeds, and/or a handful of dulse flakes.

SALAD: THE BREAKFAST OF CHAMPIONS

Believe it or not, salad is one of my favorite breakfast foods. I'm not trying to "be good"; it's just what I wake up wanting to eat. Ever since I went raw, when I wake up my taste buds wake up, too, and the coffee and baked goods just don't do it for me anymore. I want real food for breakfast—make it a salad, please. Now that's what I call a breakfast of champions!

tatiana's radish, avocado, and scallion salad

{ SERVES 2 }

2 radishes, thinly sliced

1 avocado, halved, pitted, flesh scooped out, and chopped

2 tablespoons cold-pressed extra-virgin olive oil

About 2 teaspoons fresh lemon juice

Sea salt

¼ cup Radish Leaf Pesto (see page 166)

2 scallions, white and green parts, minced

Radishes were never a favorite of mine—that is, until my boyfriend's mother, Tatiana, served me this simple three-ingredient salad. The synergy of the radishes, avocado, and scallions is pure magic. Never one to waste food, I make a pesto with the greens of the radishes and spoon it on top as the crowning touch.

Line each salad plate with the radishes and top with the avocado. Drizzle with the oil and lemon juice and sprinkle with salt. Spoon small dollops of pesto over the plates and scatter the scallions over all.

{ variation }
If your radish leaves aren't fresh enough to make into pesto, try one of my other pestos (pages 166 to 167) to spoon on top.

pass the butter . . . and the radishes

When it comes to radishes, we don't usually see beyond salad, but the French do—they serve them simply with a little butter and salt. Raw butter isn't easily available, so when you get your hands on some, make sure to stop at the supermarket on the way home to pick up a bunch of radishes.

fennel and radicchio salad
WITH RASPBERRY VINAIGRETTE

{ SERVES 4 }

2 small fennel bulbs

2 small heads radicchio, torn into bite-size pieces

¼ cup fresh mint leaves, cut into chiffonade (see below)

Raspberry Vinaigrette (page 126)

½ cup raspberries

¼ cup raw sunflower seeds

Thin slices of raw goat's milk Brie cheese, such as Blue Ledge Farm, for serving (optional)

Sweet and juicy raspberries, bitter radicchio, crisp fennel, and rich and creamy Brie—the flavors and textures play off each other and delight the senses. And then the salad gets dressed up in pink with a raspberry vinaigrette to make it simply gorgeous to look at.

To prepare the fennel, cut off the stalks from the top of the bulb, removing and reserving the feathery fronds. Remove any tough or discolored leaves. Cut the bulb into quarters, remove the inner core, and thinly slice the quarters in the direction of the grain. Chop the fronds and set aside for the garnish.

In a serving bowl, combine the sliced fennel bulb, radicchio, and mint. Toss the salad with enough dressing to coat, reserving a little to finish the dish.

Spoon into salad bowls and top with the raspberries, sunflower seeds, reserved fennel fronds, and cheese, if using. Drizzle with as much of the remaining dressing as you like.

{ how to cut into chiffonade }

This is a method of cutting herbs or other greens into long, ribbonlike strips. It looks pretty and adds a touch of style to your presentation. Try it out on basil, spinach, collard greens, and chard as well.
How to chiffonade:

1. Remove the stems from your herb or leafy vegetable.

2. Gently and evenly stack a few leaves lengthwise in front of you.

3. Using your fingertips, take hold of the edge of the stack closest to you and roll up the leaves into a tightly bundled cigar shape.

4. Use a sharp knife to cut the bundle crosswise into thin, even slices, and then gently separate the strips.

broccoli and carrot salad

{ SERVES 4 }

1 large head broccoli (about 1¼ pounds), broken into tiny florets

1 large carrot, shredded on the large holes of a box grater

½ medium red onion, finely chopped

2 scallions, white and green parts, finely chopped

¼ cup chopped raw black olives

dressing

½ cup cold-pressed olive oil or Udo's Choice Oil Blend (see page 58)

1 tablespoon raw apple cider vinegar

1 to 2 tablespoons fresh lime juice, to taste

1 tablespoon nutritional yeast

1 teaspoon sea salt

¼ teaspoon freshly ground black pepper

Pinch of cayenne pepper

1 medium tomato, seeded and chopped

¼ cup raw sunflower seeds

Massage and marinate. That's the secret to tenderizing broccoli without cooking it—massage the dressing into the florets and marinate them a bit to soften them. Two other reasons to eat your broccoli raw: It retains its vibrant green color (unlike the gray boiled broccoli I knew as a teenager) and it keeps longer without getting soggy. Not to mention the amazing cancer-preventive benefits of raw broccoli you wouldn't want to miss (see page 144).

....

In a large bowl, combine the broccoli, carrot, onion, scallions, and olives.

In a small separate bowl, whisk together the dressing ingredients. Pour the dressing over the broccoli mixture and stir well to coat. Then use your clean hands to massage the dressing into the salad.

Add the tomato and stir. Cover and refrigerate for at least 1 hour or overnight.

Spoon into bowls, sprinkle with the sunflower seeds, and serve.

{ variation }

Substitute parsnip for the carrot.

BROCCOLI TIPS

1. Break the broccoli into tiny florets rather than chop it (chopping it tends to break it apart and cause it to crumble).

2. Don't compost the stalks: Peel their tough outer layer to reveal a hidden tender and tasty morsel.

3. Don't forget to use the leaves, as they are the most nutrition-packed part of the vegetable.

kale and avocado salad

WITH DULSE AND HEMP SEEDS

{ SERVES 2 }

1 bunch kale, stems removed (see Note) and chopped

¼ cup Easiest Umeboshi Vinaigrette (page 124)

1 avocado, halved, pitted, flesh scooped out, and chopped

1 medium tomato, seeded and chopped

½ small red onion, finely chopped

1 large carrot, grated

½ cup dulse fronds, cut or torn into pieces

3 tablespoons hemp seeds

I never thought to eat kale raw before I went raw—now I seek it out. Kale makes a hearty winter salad that won't wilt like delicate lettuce can. It may be a little tough, but chop it up nicely (everything but the stems—save them for juicing) and massage it with some dressing, and it will soften right up. Chop your kale by hand or pulse it in two batches in a food processor.

In a large bowl, combine the kale and vinaigrette. Use your clean hands to massage the vinaigrette into the kale for a minute or two to soften it. You can do this a few hours ahead, and refrigerate until ready to use.

Add the avocado and gently massage it in so some of it melts into a creamy dressing with some chunks remaining. Stir in the tomato, onion, carrot, and dulse, and then stir in the hemp seeds.

NOTE: To stem kale, fold each leaf in half lengthwise, vein-side out, and pull up on the stem with one hand while holding the folded leaf closed with the other hand.

a sprinkle of dulse

Dulse is a great addition to just about any salad, soup, or entree; it's packed with minerals and adds a distinctive salty taste that some even liken to bacon. Just buy a shaker of dulse flakes from your natural foods store and sprinkle away.

salty cucumber and wakame salad

1 long seedless
cucumber, peeled,
seeded, and chopped

1 teaspoon sea salt

¼ cup dried wakame
seaweed

2 tablespoons fresh
lime juice

1 tablespoon raw honey
or agave nectar

1 tablespoon raw
unhulled sesame seeds

2 tablespoons finely
chopped fresh mint

tip

Sprinkle some seeds—
sunflower, hemp, flax,
sesame, or Sesame Salt
(page 106)—over any
salad for some added
crunch and health
value. Or sprinkle some
nutritional yeast to add
a cheesy flavor without
the dairy.

Wakame is a sea vegetable filled with minerals, particularly calcium. Even if you think you haven't eaten it, you probably have if you've ever ordered miso soup from a Japanese restaurant. The flavor can be a bit "fishy" for some; soaking it in water and seasoning with lime tempers that fishiness. To prepare wakame, use kitchen shears to cut it into small pieces—it will expand a lot when it's soaked—and remove the thick stem after soaking.

Place the cucumber in a colander and sprinkle it with the salt. Set aside for 30 minutes, then squeeze the cucumber pieces to drain some of the liquid. Place in a bowl.

In a separate bowl, soak the wakame in cold water until softened, about 10 minutes. Remove the ribs from the wakame. Add to the cucumber, then add the lime juice and honey and toss to coat. Add the sesame seeds and toss, then add the mint and toss again.

{ variation }

Cut an orange into segments and add it to the salad before you add the sesame seeds.

watermelon and feta salad

{ **SERVES 4** }

½ medium red onion, cut into thin half-moons

2 tablespoons cold-pressed extra-virgin olive oil

Juice of 2 limes

4 cups seedless watermelon cut into ½-inch cubes

½ cup chopped fresh mint

Sea salt and lots of freshly ground black pepper

4 ounces crumbled raw feta cheese

tip

For simple summer hors d'oeuvres for a party, spear alternating cubes of watermelon and feta on cocktail sticks.

Watermelon and feta may seem like unlikely salad partners, but try it and you'll see—the combination of sweet, tangy, salty, and peppery will take off in your mouth! It's so satisfying and refreshing that it just may become your top summer salad. For a fancy presentation, use a melon baller to scoop out the watermelon, or as a variation, try tossing in a handful of sliced kalamata olives.

Note that this salad is best served right after it's made. Otherwise, the watermelon will become soggy. Have all the ingredients prepped and ready to go in advance, and then toss them together at the last minute.

In a large bowl, combine the onion, oil, and lime juice. Add the watermelon and mint and toss again. Season with salt and pepper, and then lightly toss with the cheese. Serve immediately.

soups

When I'm at a restaurant, I'm often asked "Are you eating raw right now?" When I say yes, people frequently ask me about soup! I tell them that raw soups can be more satisfying than cooked soups—it's all about the flavor.

If you're new to raw and you're not sure which recipes to start with, it doesn't get much easier than soup. Since most soups are made right in the blender, they are simple to make and there is little cleanup. Serve your soup with some crackers or bread (pages 216 to 221) and a salad to complete your meal.

tomato and corn soup with basil

{ SERVES 2 TO 3 }

1 cup fresh or thawed frozen corn kernels (see page 113)

2 large tomatoes, seeded and chopped

1 cup water

2 tablespoons cold-pressed extra-virgin olive oil, plus more for drizzling

1 garlic clove

3 tablespoons fresh lime juice

¾ teaspoon sea salt, plus more for sprinkling

Pinch of freshly ground black pepper, plus more for sprinkling

1 teaspoon grated lime zest

¼ cup finely chopped fresh basil, plus basil leaves for garnish

Earlier I told you that I often don't care for tomatoes. I should have added—except for this soup. Nothing says summer more to me than this trio of tomatoes, corn, and basil. And if you stock your freezer with tomatoes and corn to extend the season, you can make this soup any time of year. (See page 95 for how to freeze tomatoes.) Serve immediately, or chill for a refreshingly cold soup or heat in the dehydrator for a warming winter soup.

In a high-speed blender, combine all the ingredients except the lime zest and basil and blend until smooth. Add the lime zest and basil and blend briefly to incorporate.

Pour the soup into bowls and drizzle each serving with oil. Sprinkle with a few grains of salt and a grind of pepper, and garnish with a basil leaf.

A NICE BOWL OF WARM SOUP

Raw soup doesn't have to be cold—you can keep to raw and still enjoy a warming soup on a cold fall or winter evening. Some tips:

1. Warm the bowls in the dehydrator for a few minutes before serving your soup.

2. Warm your soup in the dehydrator at 115°F for 30 minutes or so before serving.

3. Heat your soup on the stovetop until it is warm to the touch or until an instant-read thermometer reaches about 110°F.

my shortcut to heaven soup

{ **SERVES 2 TO 3** }

½ cup raw pumpkin
seeds, soaked (see
page 38)

2 cups water

1 long seedless
cucumber, peeled,
or 2 medium regular
cucumbers, peeled
and seeded

1 red bell pepper,
cored, seeded, and
chopped

1 medium tomato

3 garlic cloves

2 tablespoons fresh
lime juice

1 teaspoon ground
cumin

1 teaspoon dried
oregano

⅛ teaspoon cayenne
pepper, or to taste

1 teaspoon sea salt

Cold-pressed extra-
virgin olive oil for
drizzling

David Jubb, of the former Jubb's Longevity raw food store in New
York City, contributed a vegetable soup recipe for my first book,
Eating in the Raw. It was called Seventh Heaven Soup, and it quickly
became my all-time favorite. In the breezy spirit of this book, I've
come up with a simplified version—with a Mexican twist—that's
every bit as satisfying. Top with avocado slices for a heartier dish.

In a high-speed blender, combine all the ingredients except the
oil and blend until smooth. Spoon into soup bowls, drizzle with
oil, and serve.

a quick chill for a hot day

When it's the middle of the summer and you need your soup
chilled now rather than later, simply decrease the amount of
liquid in the recipe a little, toss in a few ice cubes or some
crushed ice, and stir until it melts.

creamy broccoli soup

{ SERVES 2 }

1 cup broccoli florets

2 cups water, plus more if needed

½ cup raw cashews, soaked (see page 38)

1 avocado, pitted and chopped

2 garlic cloves

2 tablespoons cold-pressed extra-virgin olive oil

2 tablespoons fresh lime juice

1 tablespoon raw agave nectar

1 tablespoon nutritional yeast

1 teaspoon sea salt

¼ teaspoon freshly ground black pepper

¼ cup fresh mint leaves

When it comes to raw broccoli in soup, less is more—just a little of this nutrition-packed vegetable is all you need for flavor. That works out quite nicely, because raw cruciferous vegetables are a potent anticancer food, and you only need a little to do that job as well—recent research showed lower cancer rates in people who ate just three servings of raw cruciferous vegetables (that also includes cabbage, Brussels sprouts, cauliflower, bok choy, kale, and collard greens) per month. The same effects weren't found in those who ate their vegetables cooked.

So next week, try my Broccoli and Carrot Salad (page 136) and the week after, my Kale and Avocado Salad (page 137), and you're good to go!

In a high-speed blender, combine all the ingredients except the mint and blend until smooth, adding more water if needed to reach the desired thickness. Add the mint and pulse to combine.

Serve immediately, or refrigerate and serve cold.

timesaver
Pick up a package of precut broccoli florets at the supermarket to make your soup prep that much quicker.

gingery squash and coconut noodle soup

{ SERVES 4 }

2 young coconuts

4-inch piece fresh lemongrass, or 3 kaffir lime leaves (see page 159), ribs removed

1-inch piece fresh ginger, peeled and chopped

2 cups peeled and seeded cubed squash, such as delicata or butternut (about 8 ounces peeled and seeded)

½ cup raw cashews, soaked (see page 38)

1 tablespoon fish sauce, or 2 teaspoons nama shoyu

2 tablespoons fresh lime juice

¼ teaspoon ground turmeric

Pinch of cayenne pepper

¼ cup chopped fresh cilantro

¼ cup chopped fresh mint

2 shallots, thinly sliced

1 Thai bird chile or other chile, sliced (optional)

With their soft flesh, young coconuts lend themselves to all sorts of uses, such as desserts, sauces, and noodles, like the ones in this Thai-inspired soup. It's easy to turn coconut flesh into noodles: Just scrape the flesh out of the shell using a small rubber spatula or a fruit scraper (a tool that looks like a magnifying glass without the lens) and then cut it into long, thin noodle shapes. If you really get into noodling, you might want to check out the coconut noodler—an inexpensive tool that magically turns coconut flesh into noodles right off of the shell (see Sources, page 239).

Open the coconuts (see page 61) and drain the coconut water into a bowl or pitcher. Measure out 3 cups; if you come up short, add enough water to make up the difference (if you have more than 3 cups, drink the extra or save it for another use). Remove the flesh from the coconuts. With a coconut noodler or a knife, make noodles out of one-quarter of the flesh.

In a high-speed blender, combine the coconut water, lemongrass, and ginger and blend until the lemongrass and ginger are pulverized. Add the squash, cashews, fish sauce, lime juice, turmeric, and cayenne and blend until smooth.

Divide the noodles among soup bowls and ladle the soup over the noodles. Top with the cilantro, mint, shallots, and chile slices, if using.

cantaloupe and pomegranate soup

{ SERVES 4 }

1 small cantaloupe
(about 2¼ pounds),
halved, seeded, peeled,
and chopped

1 long seedless
cucumber (about
1 pound), peeled,
halved, and chopped

Seeds of 1 small
pomegranate (see
opposite)

¼ cup raw honey or raw
agave nectar, plus more
honey for drizzling

½ cup fresh orange
juice

3 tablespoons fresh
lime juice, plus more for
drizzling

1 tablespoon beet juice
(from about 1 medium
red beet)

1 tablespoon plus
1 teaspoon chopped
fresh mint leaves

2 teaspoons grated
orange zest

2 teaspoons grated
lime zest

This mildly sweet soup makes a light, refreshing ending to a summer meal, and the cucumber provides some extra cooling power. For an added treat, top it with a scoop of Strawberry Sorbet (page 205) or turn the soup itself into a sorbet—just increase the sweetener to ¾ cup, omit the toppings, and churn in an ice-cream machine. For the best results, choose the ripest and sweetest-smelling cantaloupe you can find: The more it smells like cantaloupe, the more it tastes like cantaloupe.

....

In a high-speed blender, combine the cantaloupe, cucumber, pomegranate seeds, honey, and juices and blend until smooth. Strain through a fine-mesh strainer, pressing down on the solids to extract all the juice.

Spoon the soup into bowls, sprinkle with the mint and zests, and finish with a drizzle of lime juice and honey.

{ how to zest }

The zest of citrus fruits (limes, lemons, oranges, and grapefruit) is filled with flavorful oils that will enhance the flavor of any dish; all you need is a little to make a bold statement. A Microplane grater—a tool that looks like a little wand with very fine holes—is a handy tool for the job. If you don't have one, use the finest holes of a box grater.

{ how to open a pomegranate }

Pomegranates are filled with hundreds of juicy, antioxidant-loaded ruby-colored seeds. But how to get at them without turning your kitchen red? Here's a foolproof method:

1. Cut a small cap off the top of the fruit to reveal 6 chambers of seeds.

2. Score through the membranes of each chamber from the outside of the fruit, starting at the top, where the chambers start, all the way to the bottom.

3. Fill a bowl with cold water and submerge the fruit in the water.

4. Press the fruit down at the center, and the 6 chambers will separate out.

5. Pull the pith away from the seeds; the seeds will sink and the pith will float.

6. Remove the floating pith with your hands or a strainer, and then drain the seeds in a colander and pick out any remaining pith.

tangy live borscht

{ SERVES 4 }

1 15-ounce jar Real Pickles brand organic beets (see Sources, page 239)

1 cup fresh carrot juice

1 cup raw cashews, soaked (see page 38)

4 Medjool dates, halved and pitted

Freshly ground black pepper

Cold-pressed extra-virgin olive oil, for drizzling

2 tablespoons chopped fresh dill

Cashew Cream (page 199), made without sweetener, or raw dairy cream, for drizzling (optional)

My boyfriend is Russian and a hockey player, so naturally I had to come up with a healthy version of this Russian staple. And I had to make it an easy recipe, nothing complicated with multiple steps. Now, cooked borscht can take all day to make, what with making stock, peeling the beets, and chopping all those vegetables. My live borscht takes about 10 minutes because it starts with a jar of Real Pickles organic pickled beets—a shortcut that gives you maximum taste for the minimum amount of work. And you get all the added health value of fermented vegetables to boot.

Dish up this bold-flavored borscht in regular soup bowls or in tiny bowls as a starter to wake up your taste buds for the meal ahead (in France they call this an *amuse-bouche*).

Spoon out 1 tablespoon of the liquid from the jar of beets and set aside. Chop enough of the beets to make ¼ cup, and set aside. Reserve the remaining beets and brine.

In a high-speed blender, combine the carrot juice and cashews with 1½ cups water and blend until smooth. Add the remaining beets from the jar and their brine along with the dates and blend until smooth.

Divide the soup among soup bowls and top with a couple of grinds of pepper, a drizzle of oil, and the dill. Drizzle with cream, if using, and garnish with the reserved tablespoon of liquid from the jar of beets and chopped beets.

timesaver

If you forgot to soak your cashews, soak them in warm (115°F or below) water while you prep the rest of the ingredients. The cashews will soften enough for your high-speed blender to take over and finish the job for you.

small bites & sides

Finger food in the raw—now doesn't that sound sexy?

Variety is the spice of life, right? And that's what I offer in these little dishes. A mix and match that's something really different from what your friends are eating! Something that is really amazing and easy to do. These little dishes offer a lot of variety and are great on their own or as part of a balanced raw meal, from the classic asparagus wrapped in prosciutto, to cured fish and pure vegetarian sides. But first I'll start you off with ten great ideas for small sides or even one-person meals or TV snacks to have some fun with.

The only limit is your creativity!

drop that fork! 10 easy, breezy little starters to eat with your hands

Whether stuffed, wrapped, or rolled, what these treats have in common is they can all be passed around and eaten without a fork. How much fun is that? Even more fun is to lick your fingers when you are done!

The great part about these little lovelies is that you have options—you can buy or make some of the key ingredients. And you can also mix and match—for example, how about raw blue cheese in the cucumber cups, guacamole in the tomato cups, or hummus in the lettuce leaves? Mmmm!

1. **PROSCIUTTO-WRAPPED FIGS:** Wrap thin prosciutto slices around dried figs and place seam-side down on a serving platter. Try it with bresaola (cured beef), too.

2. **BLUE CHEESE–STUFFED OLIVES:** Stuff large pitted raw olives with small bits of raw blue cheese.

3. **CUCUMBER CUPS:** Slice cucumbers into ¾-inch rounds. Using a small spoon or melon baller, scoop out the seeds to form a well, leaving the bottom intact as a base. Fill with Tomato Ice Water (page 95) or any soup for an unusually pretty, tiny presentation.

4. **CHERRY TOMATO CUPS:** Cut a tiny slice off the top of the stem end of each tomato to make a cap. Scoop out the seeds and fill with Totally Raw Hummus (page 66) or pesto (page 166).

5. **CHIVE-WRAPPED GRAVLAX:** Cut Gravlax (page 154) into thin strips; roll up the strips and place seam-side down on your serving platter. Wrap a chive under and around the gravlax and tie a knot over the top.

6. **ZUCCHINI WRAPS:** Cut long, thin lengthwise strips of zucchini using a wide vegetable peeler. Place the strips on a work surface. Toss lettuce leaves with dressing, place a couple of leaves on the zucchini strips on the end closest to you, and roll them up. Place them seam-side down on a work surface, spear with a cocktail stick, and sprinkle with salt.

7. **LETTUCE WRAPS:** Serve any salad atop firm lettuce leaves.

8. **ENDIVE BOATS:** Fill endive leaves with Totally Raw Hummus (page 66) or Guacamole (pages 115 and 116).

9. **STUFFED CELERY:** Fill celery sticks with Nutty Butter (page 100) or mushroom-walnut pâté (page 119).

10. **SMOOTHIE SHOTS:** Fill shot glasses with your favorite smoothie and dust with nutmeg or cinnamon.

prosciutto-wrapped asparagus spears

{ **MAKES 24 SPEARS** }

24 thin asparagus
spears

2 tablespoons cold-
pressed extra-virgin
olive oil

1 teaspoon grated
lemon zest

1½ tablespoons fresh
lemon juice

1 garlic clove, pressed
through a garlic press

¼ teaspoon freshly
ground black pepper,
plus more for sprinkling

Pinch of sea salt, plus
more for sprinkling

½ cup finely grated
Parmigiano-Reggiano
cheese

12 paper-thin slices
prosciutto, halved
lengthwise

Prosciutto is a real treat for meat-loving raw foodists, as it is air-dried
and cured with no heat involved, and you can find it right at the deli
section of many supermarkets. Now you can make this classic party
appetizer while keeping it all raw! If you're avoiding cheese, omit the
Parmigiano-Reggiano.

Snap off the woody bottoms from the asparagus spears (they
will snap easily at the point where the stem becomes tender)
and discard them. Peel the bottom half of the asparagus with a
vegetable peeler.

In a large bowl or plastic zip-top bag, combine the oil, lemon
zest and juice, garlic, pepper, and salt. Add the asparagus and
toss to coat in the mixture.

Place the asparagus on a ParaFlexx-lined tray and place in the
dehydrator. Turn the dehydrator to 105°F and dehydrate for 1 to
3 hours, until softened but still al dente.

Spread the grated cheese over a large plate or baking pan.
Roll the asparagus spears in the cheese to coat them, then roll
½ slice prosciutto around each asparagus spear, keeping the tip
exposed. Arrange on a platter seam-side down and sprinkle with
salt and pepper.

quinoa and pesto-stuffed tomatoes

{ **SERVES 4; MAKES 4 STUFFED TOMATO HALVES** }

2 medium tomatoes

Sea salt

1½ cups sprouted quinoa (see page 39)

⅓ cup pesto (page 166)

Freshly ground black pepper

Cold-pressed extra-virgin olive oil, for drizzling

4 fresh basil leaves

Shaved Parmigiano-Reggiano cheese (optional)

For someone who is iffy on tomatoes like I am, I've certainly found lots of ways to use these red suckers! In this recipe, they make neat little containers for any combination of grains, seeds, and pesto, or other toppings. Use the recipe as a springboard for your own stuffed creations—perhaps sprouted millet (see page 39) with Blue Cheese Vinaigrette (page 127) or sprouted buckwheat (see page 39) with sun-dried tomato sauce (page 176), to name a couple.

Stuffed tomatoes are usually cooked to soften them; my raw setting-and-draining method is every bit as effective (see below). And when you strain the tomato flesh you've scooped out of them, you have a delectable bonus glass of fresh tomato juice—just add a pinch of salt and perhaps a pinch of celery seed—to enjoy alongside.

Cut the tomatoes in half crosswise and scoop out the flesh. Set the shells aside. Strain the flesh through a fine-mesh strainer into a bowl, pressing on the flesh to extract all the tomato juice. Reserve the juice for another use; chop the tomato flesh and set aside.

Rub a little salt into the insides of the tomato shells and place upside down on a paper towel–lined plate. Set aside for 30 minutes so the tomatoes soften a bit.

In a medium bowl, combine the tomato flesh and quinoa. Add the pesto and stir to coat. Season with salt and pepper. Spoon the quinoa mixture into the tomato halves and drizzle with oil. Top each one with a basil leaf and some cheese, if using.

celeriac carpaccio

1 small celeriac (about ¾ pound), peeled

2 tablespoons cold-pressed extra-virgin olive oil, plus more for drizzling

1 tablespoon fresh lemon juice

¼ teaspoon sea salt, plus more for sprinkling

3 tablespoons finely chopped raw macadamia nuts

¾ ounce Pamigiano-Reggiano cheese, shaved (about ¾ cup)

Coarsely ground black pepper

tip

To make this dish into a meal, serve on a bed of arugula dressed in olive oil, lemon juice, and salt.

Contrary to popular belief, you can eat most root vegetables without cooking them. The proper preparation—be it marinating, thinly slicing, grating, or pureeing—will enable you to appreciate them in a whole new way.

Celeriac, also known as celery root, is no exception. This gnarly round root vegetable probably won't win any beauty contests, but its earthy flavor (a cross between celery and parsley) and crisp texture make it the perfect pick for a vegetable carpaccio.

This is a recipe where a mandoline (see page 30) comes in handy; if you don't have one, use a very sharp knife or a wide vegetable peeler. Choose a celeriac that is narrow enough to fit in the mandoline.

Using the thinnest setting on the mandoline, slice the celeriac into rounds. Place in a bowl and toss with the 2 tablespoons oil and the lemon juice. Add the salt and toss. Let the celeriac marinate for 20 to 30 minutes.

Divide the celeriac among small plates and drizzle with oil. Sprinkle with the nuts, cheese, and plenty of pepper and serve.

{ variation }

BEET CARPACCIO: Substitute ¾ pound small beets for the celeriac.

gravlax

1 pound fresh salmon, divided into 2 equal fillets, skin on

2 tablespoons rapadura

2 tablespoons sea salt

2 tablespoons coarsely ground black pepper

1 large bunch fresh dill

Lox lovers rejoice! Gravlax is salmon cured with salt, Scandinavian style, without the use of heat. It is typically seasoned with dill and black pepper, but you can experiment with other spices such as juniper berries, fennel seeds, or coriander as well.

Serve on a platter with crackers or bread (pages 216 to 221), Must-Have Mustard (page 105), and Old World Cucumber Pickles (page 110) or on a sandwich with sliced raw cheese and Mayonnaise (page 104). Note that you will need 36 to 48 hours for the gravlax to cure, so plan accordingly.

Rinse the salmon, pat it dry, and remove any bones.

In a small bowl, combine the rapadura, salt, and pepper. Sprinkle over the flesh side of the salmon fillets, covering their entire surface. Lay a thick bed of dill over the salmon, reserving and refrigerating a few branches for serving.

Sandwich the two fillets together with the skin side facing out. Wrap tightly in plastic wrap, and then wrap it in plastic wrap again to seal well. Place the salmon on a rimmed dish or baking pan and weight down with a heavy can or the like. Refrigerate for 36 to 48 hours to cure, draining any liquid every 12 hours and turning the wrapped packet over.

Unwrap the plastic, remove and discard the dill, and scrape off any loose salt and rapadura. Thinly slice and serve with the reserved dill. It will keep in the refrigerator for up to a week.

smashed plantains

2 plantains, halved crosswise and middle string removed

1 small garlic clove, pressed through a garlic press

2 teaspoons fresh lime juice

1 tablespoon cold-pressed extra-virgin olive oil

A few grinds of black pepper

Large pinch of sea salt

We don't usually think of plantains as something to eat raw, but if you wait until they are really black and squishy—just when you might think it is time to toss them—that's when they're ready to mash for this sweet and tangy side dish. Serve alongside any main dish; it makes a perfect partner for my Perfectly Seared Steak (page 70).

Scoop the plantains from their skins with a spoon; use a grapefruit spoon if you have one. Place them in a large bowl and add the remaining ingredients. Mash with a potato masher until smooth, with a few chunks remaining.

{ variations }

COCONUT SMASHED PLANTAINS: Add 1 to 2 tablespoons shredded coconut.

MINT SMASHED PLANTAINS: Add ¼ cup chopped fresh mint.

INDIAN SPICE SMASHED PLANTAINS: Add ½ teaspoon garam masala.

pureed butternut squash
WITH FALL SPICES

{ SERVES 4 }

1 medium butternut squash (about 2 pounds), peeled, halved, seeded, and roughly chopped

¼ cup water

¼ cup coconut nectar

¼ cup raw agave nectar

2 tablespoons raw coconut oil

2 teaspoons fresh lemon juice

Pinch of sea salt, plus more for sprinkling

Pinch of cayenne pepper

Pinch of ground cinnamon

Pinch of ground cloves

Pinch of grated nutmeg, plus more for sprinkling

Pinch of ground ginger

Cold-pressed extra-virgin olive oil for drizzling

Squash is one of the many root vegetables that work perfectly uncooked. Sweet and slightly nutty, butternut squash releases moisture when it is pureed, yielding a creamy texture that you wouldn't think possible from a raw preparation. The color of cooked pureed squash is a dull orange and the texture tends to be heavy; in the raw it is a vibrant orange with a delightfully light and airy quality to it. Serve it alongside any entree, or use it as a spread for crackers or bread.

Combine the squash, water, coconut nectar, agave, coconut oil, and lemon juice in a food processor and process, scraping down the sides of the machine as needed, until smooth, about 5 minutes. Turn the machine off once or twice for about 30 seconds to avoid overheating.

Add the salt, cayenne, cinnamon, cloves, nutmeg, and ginger and process until incorporated. Transfer to a high-speed blender and blend until smooth.

Spoon the puree into serving bowls and top with a drizzle of olive oil and a sprinkle of salt and nutmeg.

timesaver
Cut your squash in advance and have it ready when you are, or buy prepared squash that is peeled, chopped, and ready to go from the produce section of the supermarket.

beets and carrots with coconut

{ **SERVES 4 TO 6** }

2 cups grated carrots
(about 4 medium
carrots, grated on the
large holes of a box
grater)

2 cups grated beets
(about 4 medium beets,
grated on the large
holes of a box grater)

Meat of 1 young
coconut (see page 61
for how to crack it),
finely chopped

½ cup coconut water

¼ cup fresh lime juice

¼ teaspoon ground
cumin

¼ teaspoon ground
turmeric

¼ teaspoon dried
fenugreek leaves
(optional)

1 teaspoon sea salt,
or to taste

1 green chile, minced,
or to taste

2 garlic cloves, pressed
through a garlic press

2 teaspoons ginger
juice (see page 93)

This fall dish with a tangy, spicy lime-based dressing is based on a South Indian recipe; I just left out the part where you cook it! Instead I marinate it to retain the crunch of the beets and carrots and bring out their sweet and earthy flavors. Thanks to Nash Patel, my coauthor Leda Scheintaub's husband, for this recipe.

In a large bowl, combine the carrots, beets, and coconut meat.

In a separate bowl, whisk together the remaining ingredients and pour the mixture over the vegetables, tossing to coat. Cover and refrigerate for at least 1 hour or overnight for the flavors to combine.

indian-style papaya salad

4 cups grated green papaya (half of a 2½-pound papaya)

1 teaspoon ground turmeric

1 teaspoon sea salt

2 tablespoons fresh lime juice

½ cup coarsely ground raw cashews (ground in a coffee grinder)

¼ cup grated fresh or dried shredded coconut

2 small green chiles, finely chopped

¼ cup chopped fresh cilantro

Peach-colored papaya is sweet and juicy; green papaya is firm and savory. Green is the type that's used in Asian-style salads that often feature lime, chiles, and herbs. Rubbing the papaya with salt releases the liquid from the fruit, giving it a pleasing crunch, and the turmeric gives it an attractive yellow hue. The end result is a salad that's tangy, salty, spicy, slightly sweet, and highly addictive—but it's salad, not dessert, so feel free to eat to your heart's content!

Green papaya can be found in Asian markets and in some supermarkets.

Place the papaya in a large bowl. Add the turmeric and salt and stir well with a wooden spoon, or gently massage with your hands to incorporate the turmeric and salt into the papaya. Set aside for 20 minutes.

Gently squeeze the liquid from the papaya with your hands and return the papaya to the bowl. Add the lime juice and stir. Add the cashews, coconut, chiles, and cilantro and stir to combine.

thai-style mango salad

{ **SERVES 4 TO 6** }

dressing

1 teaspoon grated lime zest

2 tablespoons fresh lime juice

2 tablespoons fish sauce

2 teaspoons cold-pressed extra-virgin olive oil

1 garlic clove, minced

½ teaspoon grated fresh ginger

2 or 3 kaffir lime leaves (see below), ground into a powder using a mortar and pestle (optional)

¼ teaspoon red chile flakes

salad

2 green mangos

1 medium red bell pepper, cored, seeded, and cut into thin strips

1 medium carrot, coarsely grated

1 shallot, thinly sliced

2 scallions, green and white parts, thinly sliced

⅓ cup chopped raw cashews

½ cup chopped fresh cilantro

Large lettuce leaves, for serving

Mung bean sprouts, for serving (optional)

This recipe is based on a salad that my Raw Essentials (www.RawEssentials.com) skin care team fell in love with in a restaurant outside Toronto. If you fall in love with it, too, to make your life easier you might want to invest in a clever little gadget called the Pro-Slice Thai Peeler. It's shaped like a regular peeler but has a zig-zag blade that shreds your mango (or papaya or any other firm fruit) quickly and in a most attractive fashion, just like they do at your neighborhood Thai restaurant. You can find the Thai Peeler in Asian markets or online (see Sources, page 239).

Vegetarians can omit the fish sauce.

To make the dressing, in a medium bowl, whisk together the lime zest and juice and the fish sauce. Gradually whisk in the oil until emulsified. Whisk in the garlic, ginger, ground lime leaves, if using, and red chile flakes. Set aside.

To make the salad, peel the mangos, cut the flesh away from the pits, and then cut the flesh into thin julienne strips or coarsely grate it. Place the mango in a large bowl and add the bell pepper, carrot, shallot, scallions, and cashews. Toss until combined. Add the dressing and toss to coat. Add the cilantro and toss again. Serve on a bed of lettuce and top with sprouts, if using.

KAFFIR LIME LEAVES

The kaffir lime is a small, gnarly-looking lime grown in Southeast Asia. The leaves of the fruit are highly aromatic, almost intoxicatingly so. If you've ever wondered what makes Thai food so good, it's the lime leaves—along with fish sauce—that give it its distinctive flavor. You can find kaffir lime leaves in Asian groceries. If fresh are unavailable, frozen are a good substitute, but avoid dried lime leaves, as much of the flavor is lost when they are dried.

middle eastern–style cauliflower "rice" salad

WITH PINE NUTS AND CURRANTS

{ SERVES 4 }

1 medium head cauliflower, cut or broken into 2-inch florets

⅓ cup raw pine nuts

¼ cup dried currants, cranberries, or raisins

¼ cup minced red onion or 4 scallions (white and green parts), finely chopped

2 tablespoons cold-pressed extra-virgin olive oil

3 tablespoons fresh lemon juice, or more to taste

1 teaspoon grated orange zest

1 tablespoon fresh orange juice

1 teaspoon ground coriander

1 teaspoon ground cumin

2 pinches ground cinnamon

½ teaspoon sea salt, or more to taste

¼ teaspoon freshly ground black pepper or cayenne pepper (optional)

1 cup minced fresh cilantro

⅓ cup minced fresh parsley

Handful of finely chopped fresh mint leaves

Who knew that the humble cauliflower—with a little help from the Middle Eastern spice box—could provide so much pleasure to the senses? This recipe comes courtesy of Paris-born Marie Pavillard, who has traveled the world over, working as a whole foods chef and educating people about nutrition, creative raw food cuisine, and a conscious green lifestyle.

In a food processor, pulse the cauliflower in 2 or 3 batches until it has a ricelike consistency. Take care not to overprocess it or it will turn to mush. Transfer to a large bowl and add the pine nuts, currants, and onion. Toss to combine.

In a small bowl, combine the oil, lemon juice, orange zest and juice, coriander, cumin, cinnamon, salt, and pepper, if using, and whisk to combine.

Add the dressing to the cauliflower mixture and toss to coat it well. Taste and adjust the seasonings if needed. Add the cilantro, parsley, and mint and toss.

wild rice pilaf

{ SERVES 4 }

2 cups raw wild rice, soaked (see page 39)

1 red bell pepper, cored, seeded, and finely chopped

1 large carrot, finely chopped

¼ cup cold-pressed extra-virgin olive oil

2 tablespoons fresh orange juice

1 tablespoon raw apple cider vinegar or coconut vinegar

1 teaspoon grated lemon zest

1 tablespoon fresh lemon juice

½ teaspoon sea salt, or to taste

2 tablespoons finely chopped fresh parsley or other herb

½ cup chopped raw pecans

Wild rice is not actually a rice but a member of the grass family. Traditionally it is grown in lakes and ponds and is harvested by hand from boats, though nowadays much of it is mechanically harvested in large paddies. Whether it is harvested by hand or by machine, wild rice is usually heated to high temperatures before it's packaged. A lot of "raw" recipes out there call for soaking conventional (cooked) wild rice for several days until it bursts—this may soften the rice, but it doesn't take away from the fact that it's not raw.

To order truly raw wild rice, see the Sources on page 239. You need only soak the rice overnight to soften it, and it is ready to be used.

Drain and rinse the wild rice thoroughly. Gently squeeze any excess water from the wild rice and pat with a paper towel to absorb as much water as possible. Place in a large bowl and add the bell pepper and carrot.

In a medium bowl or lidded jar, combine the oil, orange juice, vinegar, lemon zest and lemon juice, and salt and whisk or shake to emulsify. Pour the dressing over the wild rice mixture and stir to combine. Stir in the parsley and then add the pecans.

{ variations }

WILD RICE WITH CRANBERRIES: Add ½ cup dried cranberries.

WILD RICE WITH RAISINS: Add ½ cup raisins.

WILD RICE WITH SALTY-SWEET PECANS: Substitute Sweet and Salty Pecans (page 224) for the regular pecans.

the main attraction

If you put your mind to it, you can do anything you wish to do. You can make a cooked meal, a half cooked–half raw meal, or, as you will see in the recipes that follow, you can make spectacular all-raw meals. And if you are afraid your family won't be up for a raw meal, try my secret—don't tell them it is raw until after they eat it!

Whether it's a simple noodle dish for a weekday dinner; a high-protein, low-carb meal; or something out of the ordinary to wow friends and family, the recipes here have something for everyone—vegetarians, vegans, and omnivores alike.

baby bok choy

WITH LIME AND COCONUT CREAM SAUCE AND PARSNIP "RICE"

{ **SERVES 4** }

You can put the lime in the coconut and eat it all up—I promise. Bok choy is at its best in the raw, as that's how it optimally retains its lovely crunch. Here it is tossed with a silky smooth coconut sauce that you'd think was decadent if it weren't raw and filled with healthy, nourishing essential fatty acids. An out-of-the-ordinary take on rice made from parsnips rounds out the meal.

The sauce makes about 1½ cups; any remaining sauce can be saved for up to a week and tossed with vegetable noodles, served as a dip, or thinned with a little water and used to dress a salad.

To make the sauce, in a high-speed blender, blend the coconut water with the lime leaf, if using, to pulverize the leaf. Add the remaining ingredients and blend until smooth and creamy.

Cut off the bottoms of the bok choy. Rinse each stalk, pat dry, and thinly slice the stalks and leaves. If the stalks are particularly thick, cut them in half lengthwise before slicing. Place the bok choy in a large bowl and add the mushrooms. Add enough sauce to coat the vegetables and toss well. Set aside to marinate for 30 minutes.

Meanwhile, make the parsnip "rice": Combine all the ingredients in a food processor and pulse until finely ground with a fluffy, ricelike texture.

Spoon the bok choy into bowls and serve the parsnip "rice" alongside.

sauce

- ½ cup coconut water or water
- 1 kaffir lime leaf (see page 159; optional)
- 1 cup packed young coconut meat
- ¾ cup soaked raw cashews (see page 38)
- ¼ cup cold-pressed extra-virgin olive oil
- ¼ cup fresh lime juice
- 1 tablespoon raw honey (optional)
- 2 teaspoons fish sauce or nama shoyu
- 1 garlic clove
- 1 teaspoon sea salt
- Pinch of cayenne pepper
- Pinch of ground cumin
- Pinch of ground turmeric

- 6 heads baby bok choy, or 3 heads regular bok choy
- 1 cup very thinly sliced shiitake mushroom caps

parsnip "rice"

- 4 small to medium parsnips, peeled
- 1 tablespoon cold-pressed sesame oil or extra-virgin olive oil
- 2 teaspoons nama shoyu
- ¼ teaspoon sea salt, or to taste

> **timesaver**
> Make the sauce a day ahead and the parsnip "rice" earlier in the day, and keep both refrigerated until you're ready to use them.

kelp noodles
WITH TAHINI SAUCE

{ SERVES 4 }

¾ cup raw sesame tahini

¼ cup nama shoyu

¼ cup fresh lemon juice

1 tablespoon raw apple cider vinegar

1 garlic clove

¼ teaspoon sea salt

¼ cup nutritional yeast

1 teaspoon ground turmeric

1 tablespoon non-GMO soy lecithin (optional)

4 to 5 scallions, white and green parts, finely chopped

1 pound kelp noodles (see Sources, page 239)

1 zucchini, julienned or spiral cut (see page 30)

1 cup stemmed and finely chopped kale

1 pint cherry tomatoes, halved

Large handful of cilantro leaves, minced

Large handful of mint leaves, cut into chiffonade (see page 135)

Kelp noodles are a raw revelation—they look like noodles and taste like noodles but are made from seaweed. (But without the seaweed flavor!) This means they are a great way to eat your sea veggies. And as an added bonus, they are practically calorie and carb free! The noodles absorb any sauce you put on them, creating the perfect canvas for countless preparations. The sauce is also delicious as a salad dressing. You'll find the soy lecithin at natural foods stores. Use it for a smoother texture.

This recipe comes courtesy of Marilyn Chiarello, a certified raw vegan chef, educator, and healthy lifestyle coach. She is the founder of A Taste of Light (www.atasteoflight.com).

To make the sauce, combine the tahini, nama shoyu, lemon juice, vinegar, ½ cup water, garlic, salt, nutritional yeast, turmeric, lecithin, if using, and half the scallions in a blender and blend until it has a smooth and thick but pourable consistency, adding more water if necessary to thin it out.

Place the kelp noodles in a strainer and rinse and drain them thoroughly, separating the noodles to untangle them. Place the noodles on a cutting board and chop them into smaller, more or less even strands. Transfer to a large bowl.

Add the sauce and toss well to fully coat. Add the zucchini, kale, cherry tomatoes, and remaining scallions and toss well. Garnish with the cilantro and mint.

---

timesaver
Make the sauce a day ahead.

pasta pesto trio

{ SERVES 4 }

4 small to medium
zucchini, ends trimmed

GARNISHES: Chopped
fresh herbs, halved
cherry tomatoes, and/
or a drizzle of olive oil

tip

Pesto freezes very well:
Spoon it into ice cube
trays, freeze until solid,
then pop the cubes into
a freezer bag, and you'll
have individual servings
at the ready. If you have
zucchini on hand, you
can just thaw a couple of
cubes, and you'll have a
weekday dinner ready in
minutes. I recommend
scaling up your pesto
recipe when basil is in
season and freezing
enough to last you
through the winter.

I was, am, and always will be a pasta fanatic. But if you think about it,
when it comes down to it, pasta doesn't really have a flavor; it takes
the flavor of the sauce you put on it. Well, the principle is the same
here, and in the process your pasta turns into a healthy meal. Zucchini
noodles can be made in minutes, and they satisfy that urge for pasta
without leaving you with the heavy, carb-overload feeling regular
pasta can bring on.

I shared the basic concept of turning your pasta raw on page 30;
here are three fantastic pestos to dress your pasta with. The pestos
are all dairy free, but if you prefer cheese in your pesto, omit the miso
and add ¼ to ½ cup grated Parmigiano-Reggiano cheese. The pestos
all yield about 1½ cups; any remaining pesto can be saved for up to a
week or frozen (see Tip).

Zucchini noodles are a favorite with raw foodists, but you needn't
limit yourself to zucchini: Almost any firm vegetable can be cut into
noodles. Try butternut squash, cucumber, jícama, rutabaga, and sweet
potatoes.

radish leaf pesto

2 garlic cloves, peeled

Leaves from 1 bunch
basil

Leaves from 1 bunch
radishes

¾ cup raw pine nuts

1 tablespoon
unpasteurized white
miso

¼ cup fresh lemon
juice, or to taste

¼ teaspoon sea salt,
or to taste

¼ teaspoon freshly
ground black pepper

½ cup cold-pressed
extra-virgin olive oil

olive and walnut pesto

3 garlic cloves, peeled

Leaves from 1 bunch
basil

¼ cup chopped fresh
parsley

¾ cup raw walnut
halves

⅔ cup chopped raw
green olives

3 tablespoons fresh
lemon juice, or to
taste

Sea salt (optional)

¼ teaspoon freshly
ground black pepper

½ cup cold-pressed
extra-virgin olive oil

pumpkin seed and cilantro pesto

2 garlic cloves, peeled

1 bunch cilantro (leaves and stems), chopped

½ cup raw pumpkin seeds

1 small green chile, seeded and chopped (optional)

1 medium tomato, seeded and chopped (or keep the seeds for a thinner sauce)

2 tablespoons unpasteurized white miso

2 tablespoons fresh lime juice, or to taste

Sea salt (optional)

½ cup cold-pressed extra-virgin olive oil

Using a spiralizer or mandoline, cut the zucchini into spaghetti or ribbon noodles. Alternatively, use a vegetable peeler to cut the zucchini into wide strips, and then cut with a knife into julienne strips for spaghetti or wider strips for ribbon noodles. Place them in a bowl. If you have the time, leave the noodles in the bowl, as is, to "cure" for 6 to 8 hours—this improves the texture of the noodles. Blot with paper towels to remove some of the moisture.

To make any of the three pestos, with the motor of the food processor running, drop the garlic through the hole in the top to mince it. Add the remaining ingredients except the oil and process to combine. With the motor running, drizzle the oil through the hole in the top and process until smooth. Taste and add more lemon or lime juice and/or salt if needed.

Add enough sauce to the zucchini to fully coat and toss well. Spoon into bowls, top with your garnishes, and serve.

yellow squash fettuccine

WITH CREAMY PINE NUT ALFREDO, LEMON BASIL, AND GREEN OLIVES

{ **SERVES 2** }

alfredo sauce

1½ cups raw pine nuts, soaked in water for 1 hour and drained

3 tablespoons cold-pressed extra-virgin olive oil

¼ cup fresh lemon juice

1 tablespoon nutritional yeast

½ teaspoon sea salt

2 to 3 medium yellow summer squash

½ teaspoon sea salt, plus more as needed

½ teaspoon cold-pressed extra-virgin olive oil

¼ cup raw green olives, pitted and thinly sliced

Small handful of lemon basil leaves

Freshly ground black pepper

¼ cup coarsely chopped raw pine nuts

I stopped the presses on my first book, *Eating in the Raw,* when I heard that a woman named Sarma Melngailis was opening a raw restaurant in New York City. I wanted to add her restaurant to the Sources section. Unfortunately, I got the wrong number from the phone company and it was incorrect in the book. When I went to the restaurant, Pure Food and Wine, to apologize to the owner, out stepped the beautiful and vivacious Sarma.

Sarma has singlehandedly put the "sexy" in raw dining. Her restaurant is elegant and the food, in a word, is wonderful. I always ask Sarma for a recipe for my books and she is always generous and giving. She also sells my books at her takeout store, One Lucky Duck, around the corner from her restaurant. And she delivers her food pretty much anywhere (order from www.oneluckyduck.com). One lucky duck, indeed—Sarma is one hard-working lady!

This rich and satisfying pasta dish is made without the flour and gluten of regular pasta or the dairy, cheese, and butter of a traditional Alfredo sauce. Nutritional yeast adds a cheesy flavor and is also a great source of B vitamins. In the summer you can find fresh lemon basil at farmers' markets, but regular basil will also do fine.

To make the Alfredo sauce, in a high-speed blender, combine the ingredients and blend until smooth. If the sauce is too thick, add a bit of water to thin it. Set aside while you make the pasta.

To make the pasta, cut off the ends of the squash and julienne the squash on a mandoline or with a spiralizer. Alternatively, use a vegetable peeler to cut the squash into wide strips and then slice with a knife into julienne strips. Place the squash in a colander or strainer, toss with the ½ teaspoon of salt, and let sit for about

30 minutes so the squash softens and releases some of its liquid. Blot the squash with paper towels and transfer to a large bowl.

Add enough of the sauce to generously coat the squash fettuccine. Add the oil and toss, then add the olives, half of the lemon basil, and a pinch of black pepper and gently toss.

Divide the fettuccine between 2 shallow bowls, making tall piles. Drizzle more of the sauce around the squash. Toss the pine nuts with a pinch of salt and sprinkle over the fettuccine. Garnish with the remaining basil leaves.

timesaver
Squeeze a few limes or lemons in the beginning of the week and store the juice in the refrigerator to use in your recipes all week long.

beet and cashew cheese collard tacos

This vegan take on tacos, packed with vegetables, comes courtesy of raw chef Marilyn Chiarello, of A Taste of Light.

beet filling

¼ cup sun-dried tomatoes, soaked in water to cover for 1 hour and drained

1 cup beet pulp (from juicing 1 medium beet)

½ cup raw sunflower seeds

2 tablespoons ground chia seeds or flax seeds (ground in a coffee grinder)

1 cup grated zucchini

1 teaspoon fresh lemon juice

1 teaspoon unpasteurized red miso

1 teaspoon kelp powder

¾ teaspoon ground cumin

½ teaspoon garlic powder

½ teaspoon onion powder

½ teaspoon chili powder

½ teaspoon ground coriander

½ teaspoon celery salt

½ cup roughly chopped white mushrooms

cashew cheese sauce

2 cups raw cashews, soaked (see page 38)

1 cup water

1 cup roughly chopped red bell pepper

3 tablespoons nutritional yeast

2 tablespoons fresh lemon juice

2 tablespoons unpasteurized white miso

1 teaspoon ground turmeric

¾ teaspoon sea salt

Pinch of cayenne pepper (optional)

4 collard leaves

TOPPINGS: Shredded lettuce or bok choy, sprouts, chopped tomatoes, roughly chopped cilantro

To make the taco filling, place the sun-dried tomatoes in a food processor and process until ground, scraping down the sides as needed. Add the beet pulp and sunflower seeds and process until well blended. Add the remaining ingredients, except the mushrooms, and pulse until blended; the mixture should have some texture. Add the mushrooms and pulse once or twice to mix them in.

If you like, you can dehydrate the mixture to give it more texture: Place the mixture on a ParaFlexx-lined dehydrator tray and spread it out loosely. Place in the dehydrator, set it to 110°F, and dehydrate for about 2 hours. Flip onto a mesh screen–lined dehydrator tray, break it apart a bit, and dehydrate for about 1 hour more, until your desired "meat" texture is reached.

To make the cashew cheese sauce, place all the ingredients in a high-speed blender and blend until smooth.

To assemble, take a collard leaf and, using a sharp knife, shave off the thick part of the stem. Lay the leaf out flat on a plate. Spread some of the beet mixture on the leaf, leaving about 2 inches on the bottom without any filling. Add your choice of toppings and top it all with some of the sauce. Fold the bottom of the leaf over the filling, then fold in the sides and finish rolling to keep it together.

swiss chard burrito

WITH CILANTRO-CHIPOTLE DIPPING SAUCE

{ **SERVES 2; MAKES 4 BURRITOS** }

filling

1 cup raw macadamia nuts, soaked in water to cover for 1 hour

1 cup raw sunflower seeds, soaked (see page 38)

¼ cup sun-dried tomatoes, soaked in water to cover for 1 hour

½ teaspoon ground cumin

¼ teaspoon chipotle chile powder

1 teaspoon sea salt

¼ teaspoon freshly ground black pepper

¼ cup chopped fresh cilantro

1 large jalapeño chile, seeded and minced

Why fill yourself up on the wrap when the best part of a burrito is what's inside? When you use a Swiss chard leaf as your wrapping, you'll be treating yourself to a healthy serving of greens rather than a bunch of empty carbs and calories, and you'll get up from the table feeling energized rather than heavy and ready for a nap!

This recipe is courtesy of Doug Evans, who runs Organic Avenue, a New York City–based healthy lifestyle company known for its LOVE* (Live, Organic, Vegan, Experience) cleanses and celebrity following (www.organicavenue.com). I met Doug at the launch of my Raw Essentials skin care line—he wowed the editors from the top fashion magazines with his amazing all-raw snacks, dessert mousse, and other treats.

....

To make the filling, drain the macadamia nuts and sunflower seeds and discard the water. Drain the sun-dried tomatoes, but reserve the soaking water.

In a food processor, combine the nuts, seeds, sun-dried tomatoes, cumin, chipotle, salt, and pepper and process until smooth and well blended with a pâté-like consistency. Add some of the reserved tomato soaking water to thin out the mixture a little if needed. Fold in the cilantro and jalapeño.

To make the burrito "cheese," combine all the ingredients in a high-speed blender and blend on high speed until the mixture is smooth and homogeneous, scraping down the sides of the blender once or twice if needed.

To make the dipping sauce, combine all the ingredients in a high-speed blender and blend on high speed until the mixture is smooth and homogeneous, scraping down the sides of the blender once or twice if needed.

burrito "cheese"

¼ cup raw cashews, soaked (see page 38)

2 tablespoons water

¼ teaspoon sea salt

Pinch of freshly ground black pepper

dipping sauce

1 cup tightly packed chopped fresh cilantro

¼ cup raw pine nuts

¼ cup fresh lime juice

¼ cup cold-pressed extra-virgin olive oil

1 teaspoon chipotle chile powder

½ teaspoon sea salt

4 large Swiss chard leaves, center stem trimmed

4 large handfuls sunflower sprouts

To assemble the burritos, take a leaf of Swiss chard and lay it out in front of you. Scoop out ½ cup of the burrito filling, form it into a round, flat patty with your hands, and place in the center of the collard green. Lay a handful of sunflower sprouts in the center of the patty, and then spoon 2 tablespoons of the "cheese" over the sprouts. Tightly roll the Swiss chard leaf as you would a burrito, and cut in half. Repeat with the remaining Swiss chard leaves, filling, sprouts, and "cheese." Place the burritos on plates with bowls of the dipping sauce alongside.

peachy lime sprouted quinoa

{ **SERVES 2 AS AN ENTREE OR 4 AS A SIDE DISH** }

salad

1 cup sprouted quinoa (see page 39)

1½ cups chopped peaches (about 2 medium peaches)

2 avocados, halved, pitted, flesh scooped out, and diced

3 tomatillos, husked, cleaned, and diced

¾ cup halved cherry tomatoes

½ cup chopped red onion

1 jalapeño chile, seeded and minced

½ cup chopped fresh cilantro

¼ cup chopped fresh mint

dressing

¼ cup fresh lime juice

3 tablespoons cold-pressed extra virgin olive oil

Sea salt and freshly ground black pepper

Although quinoa has become an increasingly popular grain, I still mispronounce the name. But that's my only mistake when it comes to this salad—it's just plain great! This ancient Peruvian grain is full of protein, and the recipe is easy to make and different, too. It comes courtesy of cookbook author Terry Walters (terrywalters.net), who is at the forefront of the clean eating lifestyle movement. In her cookbooks, *Clean Food* and *Clean Start*, Terry shows us how simple and delicious it is to get on the path to eating clean and enjoying good health, for yourself, your family, and the environment.

Remember to plan a day ahead to sprout your quinoa—you can set it up before you go to bed, and when you wake in the morning drain any water that is left. Then leave it in the refrigerator until you are ready to make your masterpiece.

To make the salad, in a large bowl, combine the sprouted quinoa, peaches, avocados, tomatillos, cherry tomatoes, red onion, and jalapeño. Fold in the cilantro and mint.

In a small bowl, whisk together the lime juice and oil. Season with salt and pepper. Pour the dressing over the salad, toss to combine, and serve.

---

timesaver
Make the salad dressing up to a day ahead and keep it in the refrigerator until you're ready to assemble.

good stuff by mom & me's salad pizza
WITH TOMATO SAUCE

{ **SERVES 4; MAKES TWO 8-INCH PIZZAS** }

pizza crust

1 cup ground flax seeds or chia seeds (grind them in a coffee grinder or buy them preground)

2 tablespoons onion powder

5 cups roughly chopped vegetables (some favorite combinations are cucumber and broccoli stalk, fennel and broccoli stalk, or zucchini)

2 cups raw walnuts or pecans, soaked (see page 38)

2 garlic cloves

1 tablespoon plus 1 teaspoon fresh lemon juice

2 to 4 drops liquid stevia or 1 tablespoon plus 1 teaspoon raw honey

1 teaspoon sea salt, or to taste

¼ cup fresh basil leaves

Not only do the ladies at Good Stuff by Mom & Me have great Lemon Chia-Seed Donut Holes, which I carry on the road with me, but get this: They have pizza! So prepare yourself for a whole new take on pizza—one that satisfies in both taste and nutrition. One that has been kid tested! The two moms, Tanya Petrich and Claire Lunny, see every bite we take as an opportunity to both build health and delight our little "me"s. (See Sources, page 239, to check out Good Stuff's offerings.)

The pizza crust takes under 30 minutes to put together, but it does involve some advance planning—soaking the nuts and leaving a full day for dehydrating the pizza itself. A strategic way to go about this is to put together the crust the night before, dehydrate the first side while you sleep, then flip it, go to work, and come home to pizza night. (That will give you a crisp crust; for a softer crust, you can start in the morning and it will be ready for dinner.) You can make the sauce a day ahead as well.

Tanya and Claire suggest doubling the recipe and freezing half of the crust after dehydrating. This way, whenever you are in the mood for a pizza, all you have to do is defrost briefly in the dehydrator. If you think you won't be eating the entire pizza at one sitting, leave the crusts plain, cut them into individual portions, and let everybody top their own as they like. (Kids love the "make your own pizza" theme.) This keeps the dough from getting soggy and you can save the crust for another meal and top it on the spot.

(recipe continues)

mama tanya's favorite tomato sauce

{ **MAKES ABOUT 2 CUPS** }

¾ cup sun-dried tomatoes

1 large ripe tomato, seeded and roughly chopped

1 small garlic clove (optional)

Small handful of basil leaves

1 teaspoon dried oregano

2 teaspoons pizza seasoning or Italian seasoning

1½-inch piece fresh ginger, peeled and chopped

Pinch of cayenne pepper

2 to 4 tablespoons cold-pressed extra-virgin olive oil

2 tablespoons pitted sun-dried olives

Sea salt

mama claire's red wine vinaigrette

{ **MAKES ABOUT ¾ CUP** }

¼ cup Eden raw red wine vinegar

½ cup cold-pressed extra-virgin olive oil

2 teaspoons raw agave nectar, raw honey, or coconut nectar

1 tablespoon fresh lemon juice

½ teaspoon sea salt

½ teaspoon onion powder

½ teaspoon garlic powder

½ teaspoon dried oregano

½ teaspoon dried basil

pizza salad

1 head romaine or green leaf lettuce

1 or 2 medium tomatoes, seeded and chopped (optional)

½ medium red onion, thinly sliced

¼ cup sun-dried olives, pitted and sliced (optional)

To make the pizza crust, combine the flax meal and onion powder in a medium bowl and set aside. Place the chopped vegetables, walnuts, garlic, lemon juice, stevia, and salt in a food processor or high-speed blender and process until smooth, scraping the sides of the machine a couple of times or tamping down with the tamper if using a blender. Add the basil and pulse until well incorporated but with small bits remaining visible. Add the flax meal and onion powder and stir until well combined.

Spread out half the dough on a ParaFlexx-lined dehydrator tray in a circle about 8 inches in diameter and ½ inch thick. Repeat with the remaining dough on a second lined tray. Place in the dehydrator, set the machine to 105°F, and dehydrate for 6 to 8 hours or overnight. Flip the crust onto a dehydrator screen (remove the ParaFlexx) and continue to dehydrate until the desired crispness is obtained, 2 to 8 hours, or longer if you like your crust very crisp.

While the pizza crust is dehydrating, make the sauce: In a medium bowl, soak the sun-dried tomatoes in water to cover for 1 hour to soften. In a blender or food processor, combine the sun-dried tomatoes and their soaking water, the fresh tomato, the garlic, if using, the basil, oregano, pizza seasoning, ginger, and cayenne and blend until smooth. With the motor running, slowly add the oil through the hole in the top of the food processor and blend well. Add the olives and pulse until chopped. Season with salt.

To make the vinaigrette, place all the dressing ingredients in a jar with a lid, cover, and shake until the mixture is emulsified.

To make the salad, combine the lettuce, tomatoes, red onion, and olives in a bowl and toss well with enough of the vinaigrette to coat. To assemble, spread the pizza sauce over the crusts. Arrange the salad over the crusts, cut the pizza into slices, and serve.

good stuff by mom & me's salad pizza

WITH MAMA CLAIRE'S PESTO SAUCE

{ **SERVES 4; MAKES TWO 8-INCH PIZZAS** }

Pizza Crust (page 175), dehydrated to desired crispness

Mama Claire's Red Wine Vinaigrette (page 176)

Pizza Salad (page 176)

pesto sauce
1 garlic clove

2 cups raw cashews or pecans (not soaked)

3 to 4 tablespoons nutritional yeast

½ teaspoon sea salt, or to taste

2 packed cups fresh basil leaves

2 to 4 teaspoons fresh lemon juice

2 tablespoons cold-pressed extra-virgin olive oil

Good Stuff's pizza recipe is so good, I thought, Why limit your pizza topping to just tomato sauce? Here Tanya Petrich and Claire Lunny of Good Stuff by Mom & Me share another way to turn you on to pizza in the raw, with their fabulous nut-based pesto. As with their Salad Pizza with Tomato Sauce (page 175), the pizza crust takes under 30 minutes to put together, but you'll need to leave a few hours for soaking the nuts and a full day for dehydrating.

Follow the instructions for making the pizza crust, vinaigrette, and salad in Good Stuff By Mom & Me's Salad Pizza with Tomato Sauce (page 175).

To make the pesto, first make the cheese: In a food processor or high-speed blender with the motor running, drop the garlic through the hole in the top to mince it. Add the nuts, nutritional yeast, and salt and process into a fine powder. Transfer to a bowl and set aside. You will have about 2 cups cheese.

To finish the pesto, put the basil into the processor (no need to rinse the machine) or blender and pulse to grind it. Add the lemon juice and oil and process well, scraping down the sides of the machine once or twice. With the motor running, slowly add the nut cheese through the hole in the top until the pesto reaches the desired consistency. Save any leftover nut cheese to sprinkle on top of the pizza. Taste and add more salt to the pesto if needed.

To assemble, spread out the pesto on the dehydrated pizza crusts. Toss the salad with the vinaigrette just before serving and top the pizzas with the salad. Sprinkle with the remaining nut cheese. Cut into slices and serve.

freezing nuts and seeds

Do you plan your menus in advance? Not so much? I know it can be a little frustrating when you pick out a recipe that you'd like to make *now*, but it calls for soaked nuts or seeds. Or you set out to make your morning smoothie only to find you've forgotten to soak your almonds the night before. So why not soak a whole bunch of nuts and seeds so you always have them at the ready? Just dry them completely (a few minutes in the dehydrator will do the trick) and freeze them. Freezing does not kill enzymes—it preserves them and prevents the nuts and seeds from getting moldy. Now when you feel like making a drink, a soup, a dip, or a pizza crust, you can be spontaneous—briefly thaw the nuts and they are ready for action.

mexican layered salad

When I met Kieba, an internationally recognized athlete and life coach, on a radio show, we were five thousand miles apart—she was in Hawaii and I was in New York, and we've remained friends ever since. Kieba, whose name means "sunrise," runs an all-raw Body Temple Boot Camp in Hawaii (bodytemplebootcamp.com), where she encourages you to "start your life new and fresh, like a sunrise." Now it may be laid-back Hawaii, but Kieba loves to host and help other people become raw foodists—man, is she full of energy—and she has written four books on raw as well!

The salad is substantial enough to serve as a main dish, and the individual components can also stand alone as side dishes. There is a vegan version for those who don't do dairy or are avoiding raw eggs. Serve with Kieba's Cumin-Corn-Cacao Crackers if you like.

not refried beans

¼ cup raw pumpkin seeds, soaked (see page 38)

¼ cup raw sunflower seeds, soaked

2 teaspoons raw honey

2½ tablespoons raw butter, softened, or cold-pressed extra-virgin olive oil

1 medium tomato, seeded and chopped

1 small fertile organic egg (optional)

1 garlic clove, peeled

¼ teaspoon salt, or to taste

vegan not refried beans

1 cup raw pumpkin seeds, soaked (see page 38)

2 tablespoons raw sunflower seeds, soaked

1 medium tomato, seeded and chopped

1 tablespoon unpasteurized white miso

2 tablespoons cold-pressed extra-virgin olive oil

Dash of cayenne pepper

Dash of sea salt, or to taste

1 garlic clove, peeled

corn salad

1½ cups fresh corn kernels (about 3 medium ears)

1 small red bell pepper, cored, seeded, and chopped

¼ cup chopped scallions (white and green parts)

4 raw green olives, pitted and sliced

2 tablespoons fresh lemon juice

1½ teaspoons nama shoyu

1½ teaspoons cold-pressed extra-virgin olive oil

½ teaspoon ground cumin

Dash of cayenne pepper (optional)

2 tablespoons chopped fresh cilantro

guacamole

2 medium avocados, halved, pitted, and flesh scooped out

2 to 3 tablespoons fresh lime juice, or to taste

1 small onion, finely chopped

½ teaspoon chili powder

¼ teaspoon sea salt, or to taste

4 large lettuce leaves

Cumin-Corn-Cacao Crackers (page 218), for serving (optional)

To make either version of the Not Refried Beans, in a food processor, combine all the ingredients and process until puréed. Transfer to a bowl and let sit for 1 to 2 hours in the refrigerator if time allows; otherwise, just set aside while you prepare the remaining components.

To make the salad, in a large bowl, combine the corn, bell pepper, scallions, and olives. In a separate bowl, whisk together the lemon juice, nama shoyu, and oil. Whisk in the cumin and cayenne. Add the dressing to the vegetables and toss to coat. Stir in the cilantro.

To make the guacamole, combine all the ingredients in a bowl and mash with a fork or wire whisk until you have a chunky puree. Taste and add more lime juice and/or salt if needed.

Line 2 plates with 2 lettuce leaves each and spoon half of the Not Refried Beans on top of each. Top with half of the corn salad, followed by half of the guacamole. Serve with crackers or corn chips on the side for dipping if you like.

abundance burgers

WITH MARINATED MUSHROOMS AND JÍCAMA FRIES

{ **SERVES 6; MAKES 12 BURGERS** }

No raw foods book would be complete without a veggie burger. Thank you to Okima Wilcox-Hitt of Live Island Cafe for this one, with the works! Serve on Basic Flax Crackers (page 216), or sprouted buns, or collards, Swiss chard, or lettuce leaves.

burgers

4 cups raw walnuts, soaked (see page 38)

2 cups raw almonds, soaked (see page 38)

1 cup sunflower seeds, soaked (see page 38)

3 large portobello mushroom caps

1 zucchini, trimmed and chopped

½ large red bell pepper, cored, seeded, and chopped

½ jalapeño chile, seeded and minced

1 stalk celery, chopped

1 carrot, grated

1 shallot, minced

¼ cup nama shoyu

¼ cup flax seeds

2 garlic cloves, minced

2 tablespoons chopped fresh parsley

1 teaspoon salt-free seasoning

1 teaspoon mixed dried herbs, such as rosemary, thyme, tarragon, savory, and/or basil

jícama fries

1 medium jícama, peeled and cut into fry shapes

1 tablespoon mild chili powder

1 teaspoon sea salt

1 tablespoon cold-pressed extra-virgin olive oil

marinated mushrooms

2 cups sliced white mushrooms

½ cup cold-pressed extra-virgin olive oil

¼ cup nama shoyu

1 tablespoon raw agave nectar

1 tablespoon fresh lemon juice

TOPPINGS: lettuce, tomato slices, Old World Cucumber Pickles (page 110), Must-Have Mustard (page 105), Ketchup (page 105), Mayonnaise (page 104), sliced jalapeños, red onion slices

To make the burgers, place all the ingredients in a food processor and process until finely ground, but not a paste; there should be some texture to the mixture. Form into patties about ½ inch thick and 3 to 4 inches in diameter. Place the burgers on a mesh screen–lined dehydrator tray and place in the dehydrator.

To make the fries, place the jícama in a zip-top plastic bag. In a small bowl, combine the chili powder and salt. Drizzle the oil over the jícama and massage it in a little. Sprinkle with the salt and chili powder and massage and shake until the jicama is evenly coated. Place the jícama on another mesh dehydrator screen, and place it in the dehydrator with the burgers. Set the dehydrator at 110°F and dehydrate for about 4 hours, until the burgers have firmed up but are still moist and the fries are crunchy.

To make the marinated mushrooms, in a bowl, toss all the ingredients together and let marinate at room temperature for 1 hour.

Assemble your burgers on your wrap of choice and top with the marinated mushrooms and your toppings of choice. Serve the fries alongside.

chat

tamarind chutney

2 ounces (⅛ of a 16-ounce block) block tamarind (see Note, page 94)

½ cup warm water

3 tablespoons raw agave nectar

¼ teaspoon ground cumin

mint chutney

1 small green chile, stemmed

1 cup chopped fresh cilantro

1 cup fresh mint leaves

¼ cup water, or as needed

Large pinch of salt

3 cups sprouted chickpeas

1 cup chopped tomatoes

½ cup chopped red onions

1 cup chopped raw cashews, soaked (see page 38)

3 tablespoons fresh lime juice

½ teaspoon salt, or to taste

GARNISHES: chopped cilantro, chopped red onions, chat masala (see Note), Basic Kefir (page 90, optional)

In case you haven't noticed, I'm taking you on a worldwide tour of foods—this time we go to India! This is a raw version of a snack food found on street corners all over India. Chickpeas are the main ingredient—you sprout them here, rather than cook them—and combine them with tomatoes, onions, and cashews. Then you toss the whole thing with two different kinds of chutneys for a tangy, spicy, sweet taste sensation! If you're in a hurry, you can omit the mint chutney and just toss in a few extra mint leaves at the end. Indians top off their chat with yogurt; here we use kefir for the same effect. Omit it for a dairy-free chat.

To make the tamarind chutney, place the tamarind in a small bowl, add the ½ cup warm water, and soak for 20 minutes, squeezing the block 2 or 3 times to break down the pulp and separate out the seeds. Remove the seeds and pulp, leaving behind a thick mixture. Transfer the tamarind to a food processor, add the agave and cumin, and process until smooth.

To make the mint chutney, in a food processor with the motor running, drop in the chile through the hole in the top. Process briefly until the chile is chopped. Remove the lid and add the cilantro, mint, ¼ cup water, and salt, and process until well combined.

To assemble the chat, in a large bowl, combine the chickpea sprouts, tomatoes, onions, and cashews. Add the lime juice and salt and toss. Add the tamarind chutney, toss, and then add the mint chutney and toss again.

Divide the chat among individual bowls and top with chopped cilantro and onions and a sprinkle of chat masala. Pour over a little kefir, if using.

NOTE: Chat masala, a tangy spice mixture, is the namesake finishing touch for Indian street snacks. It contains mango powder and rock salt; its sulfurous smell is an acquired taste for some, but once you get used to it, it becomes addictive. It can be found in Indian grocery stores.

lapsang souschong wild mushrooms

WITH FRESH CORN POLENTA

{ **SERVES 4** }

mushrooms

3 cups fresh wild mushrooms, such as chanterelles, porcini, oyster, or trumpet

¼ cup brewed Lapsang souschong tea (see Note)

¼ cup cold-pressed extra-virgin olive oil

1 tablespoon nama shoyu

polenta

1½ cups raw cashews, soaked (see page 38) then dried completely

1 teaspoon sea salt

½ teaspoon minced garlic

2 cups fresh corn kernels or thawed frozen kernels

Freshly ground black pepper

NOTE: To make the tea, steep 1 to 2 teaspoons of tea leaves in 1 cup of hot, but not boiling, water for about 5 minutes. Alternatively, steep the leaves in room-temperature water in the sun for several hours.

This very special dish comes courtesy of the wildly popular raw food author Ani Phyo (www.aniphyo.com). It made its debut in November 2010 at Ani Phyo's Gastrawnomique dinner held in Los Angeles at the popular celebrity chef haven the Test Kitchen. Adopting molecular gastronomy techniques without using any of the chemicals typically used by molecular gastronomists (such as liquid nitrogen, methyl cellulose, sodium chloride), Ani created a six-course menu of raw food cuisine that tickled the palate. This dish was one of the attendees' favorites.

To create a rich, earthy flavor of cooked mushrooms, the wild mushrooms are infused with Lapsang souschong, a black tea. The mushrooms are set atop a fresh corn polenta with a puddinglike consistency.

To make the mushrooms, use a damp cloth to wipe the caps and stems of the mushrooms clean. If using larger mushrooms, cut them into smaller pieces so all your mushrooms are uniform in size. Combine all the ingredients in a large bowl, toss, and massage with your clean hands to mix well. Set aside for 15 to 20 minutes to marinate. The tea will give your mushrooms a smoky flavor, and the oil and nama shoyu will help soften them so they appear to be cooked.

Meanwhile, make the polenta: Combine the cashews, salt, and garlic in a food processor and process into small pieces. Add the corn kernels and process to mix well. Season with black pepper.

To serve, scoop the polenta into individual dishes. Top with the mushrooms and spoon over some of the marinade.

vegan bay crab cakes
WITH CREAMY DILL TARTAR SAUCE

{ **MAKES ABOUT 12 CAKES** }

egg-free mayonnaise

½ cup raw macadamia nuts, soaked in water to cover for 1 hour

2 teaspoons fresh lemon juice

½ teaspoon sea salt

1 garlic clove, peeled

crab cakes

1 large and 1 medium zucchini

1 cup raw almonds, soaked (see page 38), peeled (see page 204), and finely ground

½ small onion, minced

¼ cup diced red bell pepper

¼ cup minced celery

2 tablespoons nutritional yeast

2 teaspoons kelp powder

Don't be crabby—eat well! This recipe, courtesy of Cherie Soria, author and the founder and director of the prestigious Living Light Culinary Arts Institute in California (rawfoodchef.com), was entered into a traditional crab cake contest. It was, naturally, the first and only raw vegan crab cake ever to compete. Although it could not technically win an award (there were rules governing the amount of crab required!), it received rave reviews from both the judges and the public.

To make the mayonnaise, combine all the ingredients in a food processor and process to a puree, adding a little water if needed for a mayonnaise consistency.

To make the cakes, peel and finely shred the large zucchini. Use 1½ cups for this recipe. Peel and spiralize the medium zucchini and use 1 cup for this recipe. Roughly chop the shredded and spiraled zucchini (so the strands are small enough to form into cakes), pat dry with paper towels, and place in a large bowl. Add the almonds and toss gently just to combine. In a separate bowl, combine the onion, bell pepper, and celery. Add to the zucchini mixture, and then add the nutritional yeast and kelp powder and toss again lightly just to combine. Handle the mixture gently so it does not break down. Carefully add the mayonnaise to the mixture and toss to blend in the mayonnaise. Handle it gently so it does not become packed together.

Using a ¼-cup measuring cup, create small cakes about ¾ inch thick and place them on a mesh screen–lined dehydrator tray, with the smooth side facing up. Place in the dehydrator, set it to 135°F (see Note), and dehydrate for 2 hours. Then reduce the temperature to 105°F and continue dehydrating for another 2 hours, until slightly crisp on top and moist inside.

¼ cup raw cashews, soaked (see page 38)

¼ cup raw pine nuts

2 tablespoons fresh lemon juice

1½ tablespoons raw agave nectar

½ teaspoon sea salt

3 tablespoons minced fresh dill

¼ cup capers

¼ cup minced celery

1 tablespoon grated fresh horseradish

1½ tablespoons minced red onion

While the cakes are in the dehydrator, make the tartar sauce: In a high-speed blender or food processor, combine the cashews, pine nuts, lemon juice, agave, and salt and add just enough water, 2 to 3 tablespoons, to form a thick, smooth cream with a satiny sheen. Transfer to a bowl and stir in the remaining ingredients.

Serve the crab-free cakes warm, with a generous dollop of tartar sauce.

NOTE: This temperature will not be too hot to destroy the nutrients and enzymes, as the cakes are very high in moisture, which will keep their internal temperature lower.

raw is for athletes

My boyfriend, Alexei, who is a professional hockey player, is the perfect case study. When I first met him, he ate more than anyone I'd ever known. For lunch a group of us would go out: steak, chicken, pasta, rice, and soup would appear—and that was just for Alexei. Then he'd order two or three desserts.

I wouldn't say anything; I would just watch. For six months I watched. Then one day he looked at me and said, "You have so much energy, and you always have so many instructions for the waiters. What is your secret?" After I explained, right there and then he went raw. And his seven-course-meal days became a thing of the past. Now a typical lunch will include a seared piece of grass-fed steak, a few slices of raw cheese, and a big old salad with avocado and a slice of sprouted bread. His body became a more efficient machine—as long as it's getting high-quality raw foods, it needs much less quantity for him to be at his best on the ice.

chinese broccoli in garlic soy sauce

{ **SERVES 2 TO 3** }

4 Medjool dates, halved and pitted

1 large garlic clove

1 1-inch piece ginger

2 tablespoons nama shoyu

1 tablespoon cold-pressed extra-virgin olive oil

¼ teaspoon sea salt

1 cup water

1 bunch Chinese broccoli, ends trimmed, and chopped

¼ cup sliced raw almonds

I always like to tell the story of how I came back to New York from LA after I had turned raw, and I feared that I would starve in New York. I thought LA was the place to be to be raw—even if I was making all my own dishes out there. But I hadn't even been in town long enough to buy a couch when the phone on the floor rang. It was the *New York Post* asking me to take a photo at a raw restaurant. A raw restaurant? There was such a thing? Yes, there was—Quintessence— and the owner was Raw Chef Dan. Dan introduced me to my first raw sandwich; now my life was complete.

When it comes to dehydrator dishes, Dan is a master, as this raw stir-fry-style dish shows: It is tasty and is a relative quickie—just minutes of prep time and only 3 hours in the dehydrator. Dates provide a bit of sweetness—a healthier alternative to the sugar that sneakily makes its way into many Asian dishes. You can find Chinese broccoli in Asian markets; if it's unavailable, this recipe also works well with regular broccoli, bok choy, or fresh chives. Serve this with a sprouted grain or vegetable noodles to complete your meal if you like.

In a high-speed blender or food processor, combine the dates, garlic, ginger, nama shoyu, oil, salt, and water and blend until smooth. Transfer to a bowl and toss with the Chinese broccoli for a couple of minutes to thoroughly coat it.

Place the broccoli on a ParaFlexx-lined dehydrator tray, place in the dehydrator, and dehydrate at 95°F for about 3 hours, until slightly softened but still crunchy. Serve topped with the sliced almonds.

timesaver
Make the sauce a few hours or a day ahead.

spinach herb casserole

{ SERVES 8 }

mashed cauliflower

½ head cauliflower, broken into small florets

1 cup raw pine nuts

2 tablespoons raw coconut oil

½ teaspoon sea salt

2 teaspoons chopped fresh sage

1 teaspoon chopped fresh rosemary

½ red bell pepper, cored, seeded, and finely chopped

½ medium white onion, finely chopped

pine nut cream–spinach topping

1 cup pine nuts

¼ cup cold-pressed extra-virgin olive oil

¼ cup water

1 garlic clove

1 teaspoon sea salt

3 cups finely chopped spinach (about 6 ounces, or 1 bunch)

Here is raw comfort food at its best; this casserole makes a perfect fall weeknight dish. It's easy to put together and it can be made ahead. Warm it briefly before serving for the full comfort effect.

This is another recipe courtesy of teacher, entrepreneur, and creative food technician Raw Chef Dan, who is now traveling around the world helping others to open raw restaurants and to create fabulous dishes.

To make the mashed cauliflower, in a food processor, combine all the ingredients and process until mostly smooth, with a few chunks remaining. Spread out the mixture evenly in a 9 x 9-inch glass casserole dish.

In a small bowl, combine the bell pepper and onion and scatter them evenly over the cauliflower layer.

To make the topping, in a blender or food processor, combine all the ingredients except the spinach and blend or process until smooth. Transfer to a bowl and stir in the spinach. Spread the topping over the casserole, cover, and refrigerate until chilled and firm, about 4 hours or overnight.

Cut the casserole into serving portions, and then leave it out for a while so it can come to room temperature. Or warm the servings in the dehydrator at 115°F for about 30 minutes before serving.

tuna rolls

WITH PONZU SAUCE
AND SPICY MAYONNAISE

{ **SERVES 2 AS A MAIN DISH OR 4 AS AN APPETIZER** }

tuna

¼ pound sashimi-grade tuna, minced

2 tablespoons fresh lemon juice

2 teaspoons nama shoyu

ponzu sauce

2 tablespoons nama shoyu

1 tablespoon fresh lemon juice

1 tablespoon fresh orange juice

2 teaspoons raw honey

2 teaspoons minced fresh ginger

Want to really play with your guests' heads? Serve these sushi rolls! I mean, who is to say that sushi has to be made with rice? Parsnip "rice" works every bit as well, and this dish will spark conversation. You will need a bamboo sushi rolling mat to make the rolls; they are available in Asian food stores and some natural foods stores. Make sure your tuna is top-quality sashimi grade.

First, marinate the tuna: In a medium bowl, combine the tuna with the lemon juice and shoyu. Cover and refrigerate for 30 minutes to marinate.

To make the ponzu sauce, in a medium bowl, combine all the ingredients and whisk to dissolve the honey. Divide the sauce between 2 dipping bowls.

Divide the spicy mayonnaise between 2 more dipping bowls. (You will have leftover mayonnaise.)

To make the rolls, drain the tuna and pat it dry with paper towels. Lay a piece of nori, shiny-side down, on a bamboo rolling mat, lining up one edge of the nori at the bottom of the mat. Place about ½ cup parsnip "rice" on the end of the nori closest to you, and spread it over the bottom half of the sheet, making sure it covers the entire area and patting it down with your hands, but not packing it in too hard. Arrange a quarter of the tuna over the middle of the rice in a horizontal line. Top with a quarter of the scallions and a quarter of the cucumber.

¼ cup Spicy
Mayonnaise (page 104)

4 sheets nori seaweed

Parsnip "Rice"
(page 164)

2 scallions (green part
only), cut into long, thin
strips (the length of the
nori)

1 small cucumber,
peeled, seeded, and
cut into julienne

1 small daikon root
(see Note), shredded

Using your fingers, tightly roll up the nori: Pick up the side of the mat closest to you with your thumbs and roll away from you, lightly pressing on the filling to keep it from falling off. Once you have rolled it into a cylinder (using only the bottom half containing the filling), push the cylinder back toward you and squeeze on it a little to form a tight roll. Roll the cylinder over the remaining half strip of nori (the half that's still exposed) and place seam-side down on a cutting board. Fill a small bowl with water, dip your fingers in it, and lightly moisten the seam to seal it. Repeat with the remaining nori, tuna, scallions, and cucumber. Using a serrated knife and working with a sawing motion, cut each roll into 6 equal pieces.

Arrange 2 rolls on each of 2 serving plates. Place the ponzu sauce and mayonnaise dipping bowls next to the rolls and arrange some of the daikon alongside.

NOTE: Daikon, a large white radish shaped like a huge carrot, is often served shredded as a garnish for sushi. It's not just there for decoration, though. In Japanese cuisine, daikon radishes are said to aid in digestion, particularly when eaten with fatty foods, which makes it the perfect companion for sushi rolls.

shrimp ceviche in zucchini boats

{ SERVES 4 }

4 medium zucchini, halved lengthwise

2 tablespoons cold-pressed extra-virgin olive oil

2 tablespoons fresh lemon juice

¾ teaspoon sea salt

1 pound raw shrimp, peeled, deveined, and cut into ¼-inch pieces

½ cup fresh orange or grapefruit juice

½ cup fresh lime juice (about 4 limes)

1 small red onion, minced

1 small chile, minced (optional)

½ cup chopped fresh cilantro or mint, plus more for garnish

4 lime wedges

Basic Flax Crackers (page 216; optional)

No oven required—ceviche is a form of "cooking" that doesn't use heat. The citrus juice changes the structure of the proteins in the seafood and turns the flesh firm and opaque, as if it were cooked with heat. Serving it up in a zucchini "boat" makes for a whimsical presentation. And the best part is that you can play with different juices and seasonings and add your own personal touch to the flavor of your seafood.

....

Scoop out most of the flesh from the zucchini, leaving about ¼ inch remaining. Mince the zucchini flesh, place it in a container, cover, and refrigerate until ready to use.

In a small bowl, whisk together the oil and lemon juice and whisk in ¼ teaspoon of the salt. Brush the inside of the zucchini shells with the oil mixture. Place the shells flesh-side up on a ParaFlexx-lined dehydrator tray, set the machine to 115°F, and dehydrate for 3 to 4 hours, until softened.

Meanwhile, place the shrimp in a large bowl and add the orange juice and lime juice. Cover and refrigerate for 3 hours, stirring once. Stir in the red onion, chile, if using, and the remaining ½ teaspoon salt. Stir well, cover, and refrigerate for 1 more hour. Stir in the cilantro.

Remove the zucchini boats from the dehydrator, cool completely, and fill the boats with the ceviche (you may have leftover ceviche, which you can serve on its own in glass bowls). Top with cilantro and place the boats on plates. Serve with lime wedges and flax crackers if you like.

beef carpaccio rolls
WITH SAFFRON AIOLI

{ SERVES 4 }

6 ounces organic beef filet, cut into 12 very thin slices

Sea salt and freshly ground black pepper

¾ cup cold-pressed extra-virgin olive oil

¼ cup plus 2 tablespoons raw red wine vinegar or cider vinegar

½ fennel bulb, cored and julienned

1 red bell pepper, cored, seeded, and julienned

1 small carrot, julienned

2 small bunches watercress

2 teaspoons fresh lemon juice

1 teaspoon raw honey or raw agave nectar

2 teaspoons minced fresh rosemary or other herb

Saffron Aioli (see Mayonnaise variations, page 104), for serving

Onion Caraway Flatbread (page 220) or another bread or cracker (optional)

I've always loved Italy. And in so many ways, the Italians have it right! People wonder how the Italians tend to stay so thin when they eat so much. First of all, their oils typically are cold-pressed. And many of their dishes—like carpaccio and prosciutto—are actually raw.

So here's a recipe for the meat eaters out there. In my take on beef carpaccio—very thinly sliced beef in the raw—the beef is marinated overnight to tenderize and "cook" it without the use of heat. I round the dish out with lots of vibrant greens and a dollop of aioli for a little extra treat.

Place each slice of beef between 2 sheets of wax paper or plastic wrap and pound with a meat mallet until paper-thin. Season the beef well with salt and pepper. In a small bowl, whisk ½ cup of the oil with ¼ cup of the vinegar and season with salt and pepper. Place the beef in a large plastic zip-top bag and add the marinade. Seal the bag and move the beef around to completely coat it with the marinade. Refrigerate for 6 hours or overnight.

Remove the beef from the marinade and discard the marinade. Pat the beef with paper towels to remove excess liquid. Combine the fennel, bell pepper, and carrot in a medium bowl and place the watercress in another bowl. In a small bowl, whisk together the remaining ¼ cup oil, 2 tablespoons vinegar, the lemon juice, honey, and rosemary and season with salt and pepper. Divide the dressing between the 2 bowls of vegetables and watercress and toss.

Arrange a slice of beef on a work surface. Place some of the fennel mixture at the end of the beef closest to you and roll up tightly. Roll up the remaining beef and fennel. Arrange the watercress on 4 serving plates and top each with 3 carpaccio rolls, seam-side down. Spoon a little aioli on top of each roll. Serve with flatbread if you like.

carol's dos and don'ts

DO make sure that you eat a variety of foods.

DON'T get stuck in a rut eating the same ingredients over and over again; in particular, don't eat too many dishes made with nuts or avocados, as they could cause you to gain weight.

DO eat fresh foods.

DON'T eat canned, jarred, or packaged foods that are not marked "raw."

DO think of raw food as a road to health.

DON'T think of raw food as a way to get thin; it is a way to get to and maintain your healthy weight.

DO juice at least once a day.

DON'T drink pasteurized juices in place of fresh juices.

DO drink your juice within twenty minutes of juicing it.

DON'T juice your veggies and then store the juice in the refrigerator overnight.

DO germinate your seeds, nuts, and grains.

DON'T try to germinate bottled or jarred foods.

DO eat at least 75 to 95 percent raw foods.

DON'T try to eat raw all day and then gorge on ice cream at night as your 5 percent cooked foods!

DO store your food in the refrigerator.

DON'T leave anything out to spoil—if there is any question about the freshness of a food, throw it out.

DO supplement with powdered greens— it's full of enzymes, a raw salad in a glass.

DON'T chew gum, as it uses up your digestive enzymes.

DO eat organic when you can.

DON'T think "organic" and "raw" are the same thing.

DO favor the raw greens, carrots, and sprouts at the salad bar.

DON'T fill your tray with boiled eggs, chickpeas, tofu salad, and other cooked items.

DO eat a big or at least nourishing breakfast and a small dinner.

DON'T skip breakfast and eat a big dinner; you need all your energy to run during the day. You don't need it to sleep!

desserts

This was my coauthor, Leda Scheintaub's, favorite chapter to write. She had more dessert recipes than any other kind, and I had to put my foot down. "Leda," I said, "we need to have other types of food, too!"

When it comes to desserts, going raw couldn't be easier and more delicious—not when you can eat pie, cookies, even ice cream. I promise you there will be no deprivation in the dessert department! Raw desserts won't leave you feeling overstuffed or sleepy, the way cooked desserts do. In fact, my desserts—filled with fruit, nuts, and quality oils and sweeteners—are downright healthful, so go ahead and indulge a little!

goin' on a date rolls

1 pound Medjool dates (about 4 cups), halved, pitted, and soaked for 1 hour (soaking optional)

1 cup dried shredded coconut, plus more for rolling

This is one of the easiest raw treats you can make, and these rolls are very satisfying whenever you're looking for something a little sweet. They freeze well, so you can make a big batch and always have some on hand to toss into your lunchbox, backpack, or purse.

Soaking the dates in water for an hour before processing makes for moist and light date rolls; skip the soaking for dense, firm, fudgelike rolls.

In a food processor, combine the dates and coconut and process until a paste is formed, scraping down the sides of the machine a couple of times. Roll the mixture into 2-inch logs, and roll in coconut.

DATE WATER

When you soak your dates, save the soaking water—use it to sweeten your smoothies or drink it as is in place of fruit juice.

{ variations }

CHOCOLATE DATE ROLLS: Add 2 tablespoons raw cacao powder before processing.

ALMOND DATE ROLLS: Add ¼ teaspoon alcohol-free almond extract before processing and press an almond half into each roll after tossing them in coconut.

frozen chocolate truffles

{ **MAKES 2 TO 3 DOZEN TRUFFLES** }

1 cup raw cashews, soaked (see page 38)

½ cup water

1 cup raw cacao powder

¾ cup melted raw coconut oil

1 tablespoon alcohol-free vanilla extract

½ cup raw honey or raw agave nectar

PASTRY BAG IN A PINCH

If you don't have a pastry bag, this method works just as well: Spoon the mixture into a heavy-duty zip-top plastic bag, seal it, and snip a tiny hole in one corner. Squeeze away.

Pure indulgence! These mouthwatering little bites will win the hearts of even the most diehard cooked foodists. Have some fun with this recipe and use a variety of silicone molds in different shapes: Try stars for the Fourth of July, animal shapes for kids, and hearts for Valentine's Day.

By the way, chocolate melts at under 100°F, so the chocolate itself in commercial chocolate usually is raw, but the fillers they add (milk, sugar, and wax) are not.

Combine all the ingredients in a high-speed blender and blend until smooth.

Spoon the mixture into silicone mini–ice cube trays and freeze for about 2 hours, until solid. Then pop the truffles out of the trays. Serve immediately, or place in a freezer bag and store in the freezer until you're ready to eat them.

Alternatively, line 2 baking sheets with wax paper or a silicone mat. Spoon the mixture into a pastry bag and squeeze out little mounds over the baking sheets. Place the sheets in the freezer for about 2 hours, until solid, and then serve immediately or store them in a freezer bag.

dairy whipped cream topping

1 cup unpasteurized heavy cream

1 teaspoon raw agave nectar (optional)

½ teaspoon alcohol-free vanilla extract (optional)

When there's whipped cream around, as I've always said, my arms grow as long as needed to steal it from others. If whipped cream ever goes missing, everyone knows to look in my direction.

If you are lucky enough to have access to unpasteurized cream, whipped cream is a must! Once you try real whipped cream, you'll never go back to the stuff that comes out of a can. Freezing the cream and the beaters for a few minutes beforehand makes the whipping go faster and easier.

Pour the cream into a large bowl and freeze it for 10 to 15 minutes. Beat the cream using a whisk, hand mixer, or stand mixer until the cream starts to foam. Add the agave and vanilla, if using, and continue to beat until the cream thickens, doubles in size, and forms soft peaks. If you are using an electric mixer, start on low speed, and then gradually increase the speed to high; the whole process will take about 2 minutes with an electric mixer, about 5 minutes if you beat by hand. Serve immediately.

{ variation }

CHOCOLATE WHIPPED CREAM: Increase the agave to 2 teaspoons and add 1 tablespoon raw cacao powder after you've beaten the cream to soft peaks.

cashew cream

1 cup raw cashews, soaked (see page 38)

2 or 3 Medjool dates, halved and pitted

About ½ cup water

1 teaspoon alcohol-free vanilla extract

Vegans can use this cream as you would dairy cream—as a topping for ice cream, pies, or cakes, or to make into a parfait with fruit. To change it up, try making it with Brazil nuts or macadamias. Even I—dairy whipped cream freak that I am—love, with a capital L, this vegan version!

In a high-speed blender, combine all the ingredients and blend on high speed for about 2 minutes, until thick and creamy. Alternatively, process in a food processor, scraping down the sides of the machine a couple of times—you'll need to work the food processor a little longer to get a creamy consistency.

MIXING AND MATCHING

The best part about raw is that you can mix and match. Instead of raw honey over your banana pancakes, how about cashew cream? Or a dollop of cashew cream sandwiched between two raw cookies? Anything goes!

a pair of parfaits

These parfaits use Cashew Cream as their base and are open to interpretation—try customizing the recipes with any of your favorite fruits, such as bananas, mangos, or strawberries. Nuts are full of nutrients, but they are also very fatty and there are a lot of them in here. So remember the golden rule of raw: Never eat too much of one thing, even if it's a good thing—think of raw desserts as an enlightened indulgence.

peach parfait

{ SERVES 4 }

1 recipe Cashew Cream (page 199)

2 medium peaches, pitted and chopped

1 tablespoon raw honey or agave nectar, plus more (optional) for drizzling

1 teaspoon fresh lemon juice

2 drops of alcohol-free almond extract

With the cashew cream still in the blender, add half of the chopped peaches and blend until smooth.

In a medium bowl, combine the remaining peaches with the honey, lemon juice, and almond extract.

Divide the ingredients equally among 4 parfait cups: First spoon a layer of peach-flavored cashew cream in each one (an eighth of the total per cup), then a layer of chopped peaches, a second layer of the cashew cream, and finally a second layer of chopped peaches. Drizzle with a little honey if you like.

raspberry parfait

{ SERVES 4 }

1 recipe Cashew Cream (page 199)

2 cups fresh raspberries

1 tablespoon raw honey or raw agave nectar, plus more (optional) for drizzling

1 teaspoon rosewater

With the cashew cream still in the blender, add 1 cup of the raspberries and blend until smooth.

In a medium bowl, combine the remaining 1 cup raspberries with the honey and rosewater.

Divide the ingredients equally among 4 parfait cups: First spoon a layer of raspberry-flavored cashew cream in each one, then a layer of raspberries, a second layer of the cashew cream, and finally a second layer of raspberries. Drizzle with a little honey if you like.

stuffed peaches

2 large peaches, halved lengthwise and pitted

1 ripe avocado, halved, pitted, and flesh scooped out

2 tablespoons raw agave nectar or raw honey

⅛ teaspoon alcohol-free almond extract

1 tablespoon finely chopped raw almonds (optional)

My favorite secret ingredient—avocado—gives a silky-smooth texture and great flavor to this easy-to-make summer dessert. I call it a secret ingredient because I don't like to tell people that it's made with avocado before they taste it, as they tend to get all judgmental and crazy about avocado being in anything other than salads and guacamole. If your family or friends ask you what makes it green, have them try it first, and then let them guess!

Scoop out and reserve about half of the flesh from the middle of each peach half to enlarge the hollow in the center.

In a food processor or blender, combine the peach flesh, avocado, agave, and almond extract and process until smooth. Scoop the mixture into the peach cups and sprinkle with the almonds if using. Serve immediately.

pairing cheese and honey

An assortment of raw cheeses arranged on a platter with a drizzle of honey is a simple yet sophisticated ending to any meal. The sweetness of honey complements the flavors of a wide variety of cheeses: A light honey softens the flavor of salty, pungent blue cheese; dark buckwheat honey works well with a mild aged goat cheese. I also love Parmigiano-Reggiano with pear and any type of honey. I learned about this pairing in Italy, where it is usually the first dessert to go at a party.

triple orange salad

WITH PISTACHIOS AND MINT

{ SERVES 4 }

4 oranges, cut into segments

2 teaspoons grated orange zest

3 tablespoons raw agave nectar

1 tablespoon orange flower water

Pinch of ground cinnamon

3 tablespoons chopped raw pistachios

2 tablespoons fresh mint leaves cut into chiffonade (see page 135)

It's so easy I almost forgot—fruit for dessert! When you're looking for something a little sweet after a heavy meal, you can't go wrong with fruit salad. This one—bursting with orange flavor three ways—is one of my favorites. You can find orange flower water in Middle Eastern groceries and in the international foods section of some supermarkets.

Place the oranges in a medium bowl. In a small bowl, whisk together the orange zest, agave nectar, orange flower water, and cinnamon. Pour the liquid over the oranges and top with the pistachios and mint.

maya chocolate pie

{ **MAKES ONE 9-INCH PIE** }

You may be crazy for chocolate, but the ancient Maya of Central America were the first chocolate connoisseurs—they literally worshipped it. It was a big part of their life and their religion: Their life-giving cacao trees were as precious to them as apple trees are to us. And I don't recall ever seeing any pictures of overweight Maya.

They also were fond of avocados, though I doubt they ever combined the two. They favored making a drink out of chocolate flavored with spices, which was the inspiration for this recipe. Add a pinch of cayenne pepper to make it even more authentic, or omit the spices completely for a good old simple chocolate pie.

To make the crust, combine all the ingredients in a food processor and process to form a coarse puree (don't overprocess or it will turn to nut butter). Press the crust into a 9-inch pie pan.

To make the filling, in the food processor, combine the dates with ¼ cup of their soaking water and the vanilla and process until a paste is formed, scraping down the sides of the machine as needed. Add the avocados, oil, agave, and salt and process until smooth, scraping down the sides of the machine as needed. Add the cacao, orange zest, and cinnamon and process until the cacao is incorporated.

Spread the filling over the pie crust, cover, and refrigerate for about 1 hour before serving.

{ variation }

CHOCOLATE MOUSSE: Skip the pie crust and simply divide the filling among 6 to 8 parfait cups.

crust

2 cups raw almonds, soaked (see page 38)

6 Medjool dates, halved, pitted, and soaked in water for 1 hour

⅛ teaspoon alcohol-free almond extract (optional)

Pinch of sea salt

filling

1½ cups halved and pitted Medjool dates, soaked in warm water for 1 hour (reserve the soaking water)

1 tablespoon alcohol-free vanilla extract

3 medium ripe avocados, halved, pitted, flesh scooped out, and chopped

⅓ cup raw coconut oil

¼ cup raw agave nectar or raw honey

Pinch of sea salt

½ cup raw cacao powder

1 tablespoon grated orange zest

¼ teaspoon ground cinnamon

apple marzipan pie

{ **MAKES ONE 9-INCH PIE** }

This pie, filled with healthy nuts and fruits, is a great ending to a meal, but it is so packed with nutrition that you could just eat it for breakfast. Simply put a slice in a cereal bowl, top with some raw milk or nut milk, and you'll be running strong till lunchtime. And people wonder what I could possibly find to eat for breakfast!

....

To make the crust, combine all the ingredients in a food processor and process to form a coarse puree (don't overprocess, or it will turn to nut butter). Press the crust evenly into a 9-inch pie pan.

To make the marzipan layer, combine all the ingredients in the food processor and process until smooth, 2 to 3 minutes, scraping down the sides of the machine a couple of times. Roll the marzipan into a ball and press it flat into a disk shape. Press the marzipan disk over the crust, spreading it to make an even layer.

To make the apple layer, combine ⅔ cup of the raisins and the remaining ingredients in the food processor and process until smooth. Taste and add more sweetener if you like. Transfer to a bowl, stir in the remaining ⅓ cup raisins, and spread over the marzipan layer.

Serve immediately or cover and refrigerate until ready to serve.

NOTE: To peel almonds after soaking, squeeze them between your thumb and forefinger and they will pop out of their skins.

crust

2 cups raw almonds, soaked (see page 38)

6 Medjool dates, halved, pitted, and soaked in water for 1 hour

⅛ teaspoon alcohol-free almond extract (optional)

2 pinches of sea salt

marzipan layer

1 cup raw almonds, soaked (see page 38) and peeled (see Note)

¼ cup raw agave nectar

¼ teaspoon alcohol-free almond extract

apple layer

1 cup raisins, soaked in warm water for 1 hour

½ pound dried apples (about 4 cups), soaked in warm water for 1 hour

¼ cup raw agave nectar or raw honey, or to taste

2 tablespoons fresh lemon juice

¼ teaspoon ground cinnamon

Pinch of grated nutmeg

Pinch of ground allspice

Pinch of ground cloves

2 pinches of sea salt

> **timesaver**
> **Make the crust a day ahead and store in the refrigerator.**

strawberry sorbet

1 quart strawberries, hulled

½ cup raw agave nectar or raw honey

My boyfriend loves sorbet and can eat it by the truckload. I had to figure out a way to make him happy but keep him healthy and in ice-hockey-playing shape. Voilà—this elegant but simple strawberry sorbet.

Combine the strawberries and agave in a food processor or blender and process until smooth. Strain through a fine-mesh strainer, pressing on the solids to extract all the strawberry juice. Discard the solids.

Transfer to an ice-cream machine and churn according to the manufacturer's directions. Alternatively, freeze in ice cube trays and blend the cubes in a high-speed blender until smooth.

{ variation }

ROSEWATER STRAWBERRY SORBET: The perfumy aromas of rosewater and vanilla lend a touch of the exotic: Add 1 teaspoon rosewater and 1 teaspoon alcohol-free vanilla extract to the strawberry mixture before churning.

timesaver

Make the sorbet base a day ahead and keep in the refrigerator.

one lucky duck's raw ice cream

{ MAKES 1 QUART }

2 cups raw cashews, soaked (see page 38) and drained

2 cups young coconut meat or fresh coconut milk (see Note, page 211)

1 cup coconut water

½ cup raw honey or raw agave nectar

½ cup raw coconut oil

2 tablespoons alcohol-free vanilla extract

Seeds of ½ vanilla bean, or an additional 2 teaspoons alcohol-free vanilla extract

½ teaspoon sea salt

Sarma Melngailis of Pure Food and Wine (www.oneluckyduck.com) comes through again with a wicked good recipe. Her desserts are absolutely amazing. Just try her signature ice cream—it will knock the socks off any skeptic in your family!

In a high-speed blender, combine all the ingredients and blend until very smooth. Pour the mixture into an ice cream maker and churn according to the manufacturer's directions. Store in an airtight container in the freezer.

{ variations }

CHOCOLATE ICE CREAM: Add 3 tablespoons raw cacao powder before blending.

BLUEBERRY ICE CREAM: Omit the vanilla bean and extract and add ½ cup fresh blueberries before blending.

rum raisin ice cream

{ **MAKES ABOUT 1 PINT** }

½ cup coconut water

8 to 10 drops Medicine Flower's Rum Flavor Extract

½ cup raisins

ice cream base

3 cups young coconut meat

¾ cup coconut nectar, raw honey, or raw agave nectar

3 tablespoons raw coconut oil

2 tablespoons non-GMO soy lecithin or sunflower lecithin (available in natural foods stores)

1 vanilla bean, split open and seeds scraped out

1 tablespoon alcohol-free vanilla extract

4 to 6 drops Medicine Flower's Rum Flavor Extract

¼ teaspoon sea salt

Ode to the coconut! This blissfully decadent ice cream, courtesy of whole foods chef and educator Marie Pavillard, is rich in flavor and filled with plump raisins but no trace of alcohol. The rum flavor comes from Medicine Flower's rum extract. This company makes cold-processed flavoring extracts that are totally raw—a great addition to your raw pantry (see Sources, page 239).

Combine the coconut water and rum extract. Add the raisins and soak for about 30 minutes. Drain well (save the soaking liquid for a smoothie).

To make the ice cream base, combine the remaining ingredients in a high-speed blender and blend until smooth and creamy. Refrigerate the mixture until it's very cold, at least 2 hours.

Pour the base into an ice-cream maker and churn according to the manufacturer's instructions, adding the raisins during the last 10 minutes of churning. Serve immediately or spoon into a freezer-safe container and freeze.

timesaver
Make the ice cream base and store in the refrigerator and soak the raisins a day ahead.

"soft serve" frozen fruit

{ SERVES 4 }

4 ripe bananas, peeled, cut into chunks (or chopped, if using a food processor), and frozen

tip

When you're at the supermarket and see bananas full of brown spots on sale, stock up! They might be past their prime for eating out of hand, but they're at their sweetest and best for freezing and turning into a frozen treat.

We are not done with desserts yet! If you've got a food processor, a masticating juicer like the Champion, a twin-gear juicer like the Green Star (see page 28), or the Yonanas, a dedicated frozen fruit dessert maker (see page 30), you're in luck: Stock your freezer with bananas, and when the urge hits you, give them a run through the machine and you've got an almost-instant one-ingredient frozen treat every bit as satisfying as ice cream.

To make the frozen fruit in a food processor, blend the frozen chopped banana in a high-speed blender or food processor until creamy, adding 1 to 2 tablespoons of water, coconut water, fruit juice, or raw milk, if needed.

To make it in a juicer, pass the bananas through a juicer with the blank plate in position, and, there you have it, banana "ice cream."

If you have the Yonanas, just place the bananas in it and press. Serve immediately.

{ variation }

Keep the banana as the base (it gives richness and body to your frozen treats), but feel free to include other fruit, such as mango chunks, whole raspberries, blueberries, or strawberries, or even avocado to change up the flavor.

coconut butterscotch cookies

{ MAKES ABOUT 2 DOZEN COOKIES }

1½ cups raw almonds, soaked (see page 38)

1 cup raw walnuts, soaked (see page 38)

1 cup packed halved and pitted Medjool dates, soaked in warm water for about 30 minutes and drained

½ cup raw agave nectar

½ cup coconut flour

½ cup lucuma powder

1 teaspoon alcohol-free vanilla extract

¼ teaspoon sea salt

Gluten-free and dairy-free cookies are all the rage these days—and these fill the bill. Don't miss my Turn It Raw Chocolate Chocolate Chip Cookies on page 72 to add to your arsenal of cookie recipes. You can order the lucuma powder and coconut flour online (see Sources, page 239).

Combine all the ingredients in a food processor and process until it starts to form a ball, scraping down the sides of the bowl a few times (you may need to do this in 2 batches).

Use a small cookie scoop, about 1½ inches in diameter, to scoop up the dough (don't pack it into the scoop) and place on a mesh screen–lined dehydrator tray (the cookies won't spread, so you don't need to leave much space between them). Place in the dehydrator, set it for 115°F, and dehydrate for about 24 hours (don't flip them) until firm on the outside but still a little moist on the inside. For little bite-size cookies, use a 1-inch cookie scoop.

Eat a few warm from the dehydrator because they're so good, and then cool the rest and store in an airtight container in the refrigerator for up to 2 weeks, or in the freezer for up to 2 months.

lemon "luv" cupcakes
WITH COCONUT MERINGUE

{ **MAKES 18 TO 20 MINI CUPCAKES** }

cupcakes

1 cup finely ground raw cashews (ground in a food processor)

½ cup coconut flour (see Sources, page 239)

½ cup finely ground raw macadamia nuts (ground in a food processor)

Pinch of sea salt

½ cup Date Paste (page 213)

1 teaspoon alcohol-free vanilla extract

½ teaspoon alcohol-free lemon extract

tart lemon filling

¾ cup Irish moss

¼ cup water

2 tablespoons fresh lemon juice

2 tablespoons raw agave nectar

When I met Okima Wilcox-Hitt at the Navel Expo on Long Island, she gave me a gift of four delicious, creamy, moist, lemon cupcakes—all raw, of course. Naturally, I had to go to visit her at her new digs at the Live Island Cafe immediately. And I was not disappointed!

In this recipe, Irish moss, an algae, is used as a thickener for both the filling and the meringue; you can find dried Irish moss at natural foods stores and herb stores. Make the meringue in advance if you like—it will keep in the refrigerator for 3 to 4 days.

To make the cupcakes, in a large bowl, combine the cashews, coconut flour, macadamias, and salt. Add the date paste, vanilla extract, lemon extract, and enough water to form a kneadable soft dough. Line a mini-cupcake pan with plastic wrap. Using a small ice-cream scoop, drop a scoop of dough into each cup. Press the dough into the cup and then poke a hole in the center of each cupcake with your pinky finger. Remove the cupcakes from the pan, remove the plastic, and place the cupcakes on a ParaFlexx–lined tray. Place in the dehydrator and dehydrate at 115°F for 2 to 4 hours, until a bit firm but still moist. Refrigerate to cool before filling.

To make the filling, combine the Irish moss and water in a blender and blend until the Irish moss is completely broken down and the mixture is smooth. Add the lemon juice and agave and continue blending until the filling is velvety smooth. Transfer to a container, cover, and refrigerate until it has a jamlike consistency.

coconut meringue

¾ cup Irish moss

¼ cup water

¾ cup raw cashews, soaked (see page 38)

⅔ cup fresh coconut milk (see Note)

¼ cup young coconut meat

¼ cup plus 2 table- spoons raw agave nectar

1 teaspoon fresh lemon juice

2 teaspoons alcohol- free vanilla extract

⅛ teaspoon sea salt

½ cup plus 1 table- spoon raw coconut oil

To make the meringue, combine the Irish moss and ¼ cup water in a high-speed blender and blend until the Irish moss is completely broken down and the mixture is smooth. Add the cashews, coconut milk, coconut meat, agave, lemon juice, vanilla extract, and salt and blend until creamy. Add the coconut oil and blend until it is completely integrated. Pour into a container, cover, and refrigerate so it will firm up but still retain a soft consistency.

To assemble the cupcakes, fill each cupcake hole with a bit of the lemon filling and top with a generous spoonful of meringue. Serve immediately, or place in a container, cover, and store in the refrigerator until ready to serve.

NOTE: To make fresh coconut milk, in a high-speed blender, blend young coconut meat and coconut water in a ratio of 2 to 1.

nouveau path brownies

WITH RASPBERRY SAUCE

{ **MAKES 16 BROWNIES** }

brownies
1 cup raw Brazil nuts

1 cup raw sunflower seeds

½ cup raw cacao powder

2 cups Medjool dates, halved and pitted

1 tablespoon alcohol-free vanilla extract (optional)

¼ cup raw cacao nibs

raspberry sauce
1 10-ounce bag frozen raspberries, defrosted

About ¼ cup Date Paste (recipe follows)

One day when I was home on Long Island, I walked into my favorite Health Nuts store to find that they had renovated and added a café. A young gentleman named Michael Durr approached me and told me he had read my books and had started the café to introduce raw foods to the community. He then asked me to try his brownie—at which I rolled my eyes, because so many people had tried and failed at a really great brownie. But to be polite, I tried it, and I am so glad I did. This indeed is a great recipe, born from Michael's desire to change his life and the community, and to pay homage to his friend and inspiration Eddie. Raw cacao nibs can be found in most natural foods stores.

To make the brownies, combine the Brazil nuts and sunflower seeds in a food processor and process into a powder. Add the cacao powder and process again to incorporate. Add the dates and vanilla, if using, and process until a ball forms. Transfer to a bowl and mix in the cacao nibs. Press evenly into an 8-inch square silicone or metal pan. Freeze until firm, about 4 hours or overnight, and then cut into squares.

To make the raspberry sauce, combine the raspberries and date paste in a food processor and process until smooth, adding more date paste, a little at a time, until it is sweet enough for your taste. Pour into a squeeze bottle (add water if necessary to make it pourable) and drizzle over individual brownies as you serve them.

1 pound pitted Medjool
dates

1 cup water

date paste

{ **MAKES ABOUT 1½ CUPS** }

Dates are the sweetest fruit on earth, so take advantage of their natural sugar content by making date paste out of them. Use it to sweeten any number of desserts, smoothies, or breakfast cereals.

Place the dates in a bowl, add the water, and soak for several hours, until most of the water is absorbed. Transfer to a food processor (do not drain) and process until completely smooth. Store, refrigerated, for up to 2 weeks.

dehydrator crackers, breads, & snacks

People are confused when they see me eat something that "looks like food," and I tell them that it is raw. Usually it is a pretty funny conversation because most people think that you have to use an oven to bake food.

Wrong! Dehydrating is the raw version of baking. It is baking with slow heat, and it is the only way to go when you're looking for the crunch of a cracker or the comfort of a lunchtime sandwich. I devoted a whole chapter to the subject because it is important to the enjoyment of raw foods. So before you delve into these recipes, brush up on your dehydrating basics (see page 40), and don't forget to read the manual that comes with your dehydrator!

basic flax crackers

2 cup flax seeds

2½ cups water

¾ teaspoon sea salt

I just love crackers. As part of a meal or as a snack, nothing beats a great cracker. But you can pack in some serious pounds with cooked crackers, as some of them are made with pasteurized butter, cheese, processed oils, and fillers, not to mention preservatives. Yuck!

Packaged raw crackers are a convenience but pricey; make your own and they will run you just two or three dollars for a large batch. They are perfect for snacking, dipping, or serving alongside soups and salads.

In a large bowl, soak the flax seeds in the water for at least 2 hours or overnight. The water will become gelatinous. Do not drain.

Add the salt, and then divide the mixture between 2 ParaFlexx-lined dehydrator trays and spread it out so it's about ¼ inch thick. Place in the dehydrator, set it to 115°F, and dehydrate for about 12 hours, until dry on top.

Place an empty mesh screen–lined dehydrator tray over the crackers, and then turn the whole thing upside down and remove the ParaFlexx. Dehydrate for another 12 hours, until crisp. Break the sheets with your hands into crackers approximately 3-inch square. Store in an airtight container for up to 2 weeks.

{ variations }

NAMA SHOYU FLAX CRACKERS: Omit the salt and add ¼ cup nama shoyu along with the water.

HERB FLAX CRACKERS: Add 1 tablespoon minced fresh herbs or 1 teaspoon dried herbs when you add the salt.

garlicky vegetable flax crackers

2 cups flax seeds

1 red bell pepper, seeded, cored, and coarsely chopped

2 large tomatoes, coarsely chopped

1 cup packed spinach leaves

½ cup water

2 teaspoons tomato concentrate (optional; see Sources, page 239)

2 teaspoons raw apple cider vinegar

3 garlic cloves

¾ teaspoon sea salt

Man, I do love garlic—so I make sure my boyfriend is on the road and I'm sleeping alone when I eat this garlicky number! When you want to fancy up your standard flax crackers, add this twist—and you'll be getting a bonus serving of salad with every cracker!

Combine all the ingredients in a food processor and process until well combined. Divide the mixture between 2 ParaFlexx-lined dehydrator sheets and spread it out so it's about ¼ inch thick. Place in the dehydrator, set it to 115°F, and dehydrate for about 12 hours, until dry on top.

Place an empty mesh screen–lined dehydrator tray over the crackers, and then turn the whole thing upside down and remove the ParaFlexx. Dehydrate for another 12 hours, until crisp, then break the sheets with your hands into crackers approximately 3-inch square. Store in an airtight container for up to 2 weeks.

cumin-corn-cacao crackers

{ MAKES 16 CRACKERS; 1 DEHYDRATOR TRAY }

3 cups fresh (see page 113) or thawed frozen corn kernels

2 tablespoons water

1 tablespoon raw cacao powder

2 teaspoons raw honey

1 teaspoon sea salt

1 tablespoon ground cumin

½ teaspoon cayenne powder

1 small carrot, shredded (optional)

½ cup shredded raw cheddar cheese (optional)

Kieba is one of the wonders of the Hawaiian islands; these savory-sweet crackers are another contribution from her. She is the founder of the raw-food-based Body Temple Boot Camp in Hawaii. If you want to get into shape quickly and with better health, look her up!

Serve with Kieba's Mexican Layered Salad (page 180) or pop a few of these crackers into a bag to carry around as a snack on the go.

In a high-speed blender or food processor, combine all the ingredients and blend until smooth.

Press the mixture onto a ParaFlexx-lined dehydrator tray so it's about ¼ inch thick. Place in the dehydrator, set it to 115°F, and dehydrate for 6 to 7 hours, until dry on top.

Place an empty mesh screen–lined dehydrator tray over the crackers, and then turn the whole thing upside down and remove the ParaFlexx sheet. Dehydrate for another 4 to 6 hours, until crisp. Break the sheets with your hands into crackers approximately 3-inch square or the shape of your choice. Store in an airtight container for up to 2 weeks.

what do you mean no bread?

Many people have a hard time giving up wheat. It is everywhere in cooked foods because it is a cheap filler. In addition to cakes, cookies, and bread, it makes its way into unlikely places such as soups, gravies, and baby formula. So even if you think you've given up wheat, you may in fact not be totally wheat-free.

You may be wondering how raw foodists do without bread—I mean, isn't it the very staff of life? Well, people ate wheat way back when, and they did make bread. But they sprouted their grains, though it was unintentional (grains would be left in the open air, exposed to the elements; it got wet and began to germinate before it was brought in for storage). And they ate the whole grain. They formed the batter into cakes and laid the cakes in the sun. Hey, wait a minute! That sounds familiar—isn't that dehydration?

Now that bread was, indeed, the staff of life. Then came the oven, and we started dehydrating foods faster and at higher temperatures. We traded higher heat for nutrition, living food for dead food (see page 245 for the science behind what happens to food when it is cooked).

The good news: We sneaky, clever raw foodists have reinvented bread! And in different styles and varieties, all so delicious and satisfying. Check out the recipes in this chapter, and you won't be missing cooked bread, ever!

onion caraway flatbread

{ **MAKES 18 SLICES** }

- **4 medium red onions, sliced**
- **2 cups hot water**
- **2 tablespoons fresh lemon juice**

onion marinade
- **¼ cup nama shoyu**
- **¼ cup cold-pressed extra-virgin olive oil**
- **2 tablespoons fresh lemon juice**
- **2 tablespoons raw agave nectar**
- **2 tablespoons ground caraway seeds**
- **1 garlic clove, grated**
- **1 teaspoon sea salt**
- **1 teaspoon Italian seasoning**
- **1 teaspoon dried thyme**
- **½ teaspoon ground white pepper**
- **2 cups raw sunflower seeds, soaked (see page 38)**
- **1 apple, peeled, cored, and roughly chopped**
- **2 cups ground flax seeds (ground in a coffee grinder)**

This delicious gluten-free bread comes from raw food revolutionary Cherie Soria, the founder and director of the internationally known Living Light Culinary Institute (www.rawfoodchef.com), who has been teaching raw vegan culinary arts to students and teachers from around the world since 1992. It is rich in essential fatty acids and satisfies the need for sandwich bread. Try it with nut butter, avocado, spreads, or any favorite sandwich filling. Or you can omit the caraway seeds and use it as a pizza crust.

Place the onions in a large bowl and add the hot water and lemon juice to cover. Leave to soak for 30 minutes. Drain, return to the bowl, and set aside.

In a blender, combine all the onion marinade ingredients and blend until smooth. Pour over the drained onions, massage the onions with the marinade, and set aside to marinate for 2 to 6 hours. Drain; reserve the marinade to use as a dressing.

In a food processor, combine the sunflower seeds and apple and process until smooth. Transfer the mixture to a large bowl and mix in the drained marinated onions. Put half the mixture into the food processor and pulse it until well combined but there are small, visible pieces of onion. Remove and repeat with the remaining mixture in the bowl.

Combine both batches in a large bowl and mix in the ground flax seeds.

Divide the mixture between 2 ParaFlexx–lined dehydrator trays and spread it out ¼ inch thick. Place in the dehydrator, set it to 125°F, and dehydrate for 2 hours. Reduce the temperature to 110°F and dehydrate for about 8 hours, until it's dry enough to flip. Flip over onto another dehydrator tray lined with a mesh screen and remove the ParaFlexx. Score each bread into 9 equal 3 by 3-inch squares. Dehydrate until dry on the outside but still flexible, 6 to 8 hours. Store in the refrigerator for up to 2 weeks.

live sun-dried tomato bread

{ MAKES 9 SLICES }

¾ cup sun-dried tomatoes

1 small to medium fresh tomato

½ red onion

2 tablespoons raw sesame tahini

Juice of ½ lemon

2 tablespoons fresh oregano, or 2 teaspoons dried

1½ cups water

Pinch of cayenne pepper

1 cup buckwheat groats (see page 80)

1½ cups ground flax seeds (ground in a coffee grinder)

When I moved back to New York City from LA in 2001, I had become a raw foodist, and I was happily shocked to see that the raw food movement had preceded me. Almost immediately I found Christopher Dobrowolski and Dan (RawChefDan).

Christopher runs Live Live & Organic ("live," as in the opposite of dead, and "live," as in energetic—how else do you explain how to pronounce this clever name!). It's the premier organic boutique in New York City that provides everything for the raw food lifestyle: foods and superfoods, snacks, body care products, living supplements, and more. Check them out at www.live-live.com.

Christopher is mentioned in all my books because he is an innovator and such a kind person. He runs Live Live & Organic in an effort to bring raw food to the community, and he also coaches newbies from around the country on how to prepare amazing dishes.

As raw food is not cooked, he named this bread "live." After you eat it, instead of feeling tired and ready for a nap you will feel lively and raring to go!

Place the sun-dried tomatoes in a bowl, add water to cover, and soak for 4 to 8 hours. Drain.

In a high-speed blender, combine all the ingredients except the flax meal and blend into a thick paste. Pour into a large bowl and thoroughly whisk in the flax meal.

Pour the batter evenly onto a ParaFlexx-lined dehydrator tray so the batter is about 1 inch thick, leaving a border around the edges. Place in the dehydrator, turn the machine to 100°F, and dehydrate for about 16 hours. Flip the bread over onto another dehydrator tray lined with a mesh screen and remove the ParaFlexx. Score the bread into 9 squares, and continue dehydrating for an additional 4 to 8 hours, depending on how soft you like your bread. It will keep for up to 5 days in an airtight container.

lemon bread

3 tablespoons ground flax seeds (ground in a coffee grinder)

2 cups dried shredded coconut or coconut chips

2 cups chopped pumpkin or winter squash

½ cup water

½ cup dried apricots

1 teaspoon raw coconut oil

3 tablespoons grated fresh lemon zest (from about 3 lemons)

2 teaspoons alcohol-free vanilla extract, or the seeds of ¼ vanilla pod

½ teaspoon sea salt

This is another recipe from Christopher at Live Live & Organic (see page 221 for his Sun-Dried Tomato Bread). It's sweet comfort food—perfect drizzled with honey or for making an almond butter and raw jam sandwich. Christopher's bread recipes give a small taste of what you can easily make in your raw kitchen using your dehydrator.

Combine all the ingredients in a high-speed blender and blend thoroughly until all ingredients are completely homogenized and smooth, adding a little more water if needed. Some fiber can be left coarse for texture.

Pour the batter evenly onto a ParaFlexx-lined dehydrator tray so it's about ¼ inch thick, leaving space at the edges. Place in the dehydrator, turn the machine to 100°F, and dehydrate for 8 to 10 hours. Cut into 9 squares. The bread will keep for up to 5 days in an airtight container.

"popcorn" cauliflower crunchies

{ MAKES ABOUT 2 CUPS }

1 large head cauliflower (about 2½ pounds)

2 tablespoons cold-pressed extra-virgin olive oil or raw butter, melted

½ teaspoon sea salt, or to taste

¼ teaspoon freshly ground black pepper, or to taste

1 tablespoon nutritional yeast, or ½ cup finely grated Parmigiano-Reggiano cheese

Popcorn is my favorite cheat. A hockey game just isn't the same without a bag of the crunchy, salty, buttery stuff. If you're wondering why I'm using the words "popcorn" and "cauliflower" in the same title, it's because these little crunchies have a distinct popcorn look and taste to them, but they are made from nutrient-dense cauliflower. So chow down, folks—you can't OD on cauliflower!

Note that the crunchies are best eaten the day they are made. They are extremely addictive, though, so that shouldn't be an issue; you might even want to double up on the recipe so you'll be sure to have some to share.

Remove the leaves from the cauliflower and break the cauliflower into bite-size florets. Break up the stems into bite-size pieces. Place the cauliflower in a plastic zip-top bag.

Pour the oil into a small bowl. Whisk the salt, pepper, and nutritional yeast, if using (but not the cheese), into the oil. Pour the oil over the cauliflower in the bag, seal the bag, and massage the oil evenly into the cauliflower. If using cheese, open the bag, add the cheese, and massage it in.

Place the cauliflower on ParaFlexx-lined trays and place in the dehydrator. Dehydrate at 115°F for 10 to 12 hours, until crunchy.

{ variation }

GARLICKY CAULIFLOWER CRUNCH: Add 3 garlic cloves, pressed through a press, to the oil or butter.

sweet and salty pecans

{ **MAKES 2 CUPS** }

2 cups raw pecans (not soaked)

3 tablespoons raw honey, coconut nectar, or raw agave nectar

¼ to ½ teaspoon coarse sea salt

For my previous book, *The Raw 50* (2007), my sister Christine gave me several nut mix recipes, and they were so well received that by popular demand, I've come up with a few more for this book. Dehydrator nuts have a crunch similar to oven-roasted nuts, but if you keep the temperature at 115°F, they are totally raw and you wouldn't even know the difference—cool, huh? They make a great snack for when you're on the run or to keep stashed in your office drawer. The salt goes a long way, so experiment with the lesser amount first and see what you like.

Place the nuts in a large bowl. Add the honey and toss, and then add the salt and toss again. Place the nuts on a ParaFlexx-lined dehydrator tray and place in the dehydrator. Set the machine to 115°F and dehydrate until crisp and sticky, but no longer wet, about 24 hours, turning them once.

Cool and store in an airtight container for up to 1 month.

{ variation }

HERB PECANS: Add 1 teaspoon dried herbs such as rosemary, oregano, or thyme.

curried cashews

{ MAKES 2 CUPS }

2 cups raw cashews
(not soaked)

2 tablespoons cold-
pressed extra-virgin
olive oil

2 teaspoons mild
curry powder

¼ teaspoon fine
sea salt

Fill up a bowl, pass them around, and watch them disappear. If you're having a party, double up, and while you're at it, throw together a couple of batches of Sweet and Salty Pecans (opposite) to make use of all your dehydrator trays while the machine is running.

Place the cashews in a large bowl. Add the oil and toss to coat. Add the curry powder and salt and toss again. Place on a ParaFlexx-lined dehydrator sheet and place in the dehydrator. Set the machine to 115°F and dehydrate until crisp, about 24 hours, turning them once.

Cool and store in an airtight container for up to 1 month.

chili dried pumpkin seeds

{ MAKES 2 CUPS }

2 cups raw pumpkin
seeds (not soaked)

1½ tablespoons cold-
pressed extra-virgin
olive oil

2 teaspoons chili
powder

¼ teaspoon fine
sea salt

Don't wait for Halloween! These spiced pumpkin seeds are great for eating out of hand or sprinkling on salads any time of year.

Place the pumpkin seeds in a large bowl. Add the oil and toss to coat. Add the chili powder and salt and toss again. Place on a ParaFlexx-lined dehydrator tray and place in the dehydrator. Set the machine to 115°F and dehydrate until crisp, about 12 hours.

Cool and store in an airtight container for up to 1 month.

garlicky salt and vinegar potato chips

1 cup water

½ cup coconut vinegar or raw apple cider vinegar

2 large potatoes

2 tablespoons cold-pressed extra-virgin olive oil

1 teaspoon garlic powder

1 teaspoon sea salt

What do I do when I get hit with an attack of the munchies? Like the rest of the world, I go for the chips! Have some of these on hand to save yourself from store-bought chips made with shoddy oils. They look, taste, and crunch like the real thing—now you can munch away, guilt free! This recipe will make enough chips to fill up 4 dehydrator trays if you are using the Excalibur; if you have the eight-tray model, double the recipe to fill up all the trays.

In a large bowl, combine the water and vinegar.

Peel the potatoes and slice them on the thinnest setting of a mandoline. Alternatively, use a wide vegetable peeler to slice them. As you slice them, immediately place them in the vinegar water to keep them from browning. Soak for 10 minutes.

In another large bowl, whisk together the oil, garlic powder, and salt. Drain the potatoes and pat them with paper towels to absorb most of the water. Place them in the oil mixture and massage the oil in.

Spread out the potato slices on 4 mesh screen–lined dehydrator trays. Place in the dehydrator, set it to 115°F, and dehydrate for 8 hours. Flip the chips and dehydrate for an additional 8 hours, or until crisp. Store in an airtight container for up to 1 week.

peppery sweet potato chips

{ **MAKES ABOUT 4 DEHYDRATOR TRAYS** }

2 tablespoons cold-pressed extra-virgin olive oil

2 tablespoons raw agave nectar or raw honey

1 tablespoon coconut vinegar or raw apple cider vinegar

2 tablespoons sweet paprika

1 teaspoon freshly ground black pepper

1 teaspoon sea salt

1 large sweet potato

Like my potato chips (opposite), these chips are hard to stop eating, but luckily one sweet potato goes a long way. Double the recipe to fill up all of the trays if you have the large Excalibur model.

In a large bowl, whisk together all the ingredients except the sweet potato.

Peel the sweet potato and slice it on the thinnest setting of a mandoline or use a wide vegetable peeler to slice it. Place immediately in the oil mixture and massage it for a few minutes to coat.

Arrange the sweet potato slices on 4 ParaFlexx-lined dehydrator trays and place in the dehydrator. Set the machine to 115°F and dehydrate for 12 hours. Invert each chip on a mesh screen, return to the dehydrator, and dehydrate for an additional 10 to 12 hours, until crisp. Store in an airtight container for up to 1 week.

spicy lime plantain chips

{ **MAKES ABOUT 4 DEHYDRATOR TRAYS** }

1 lime

¼ cup liquid coconut oil (warm it in the dehydrator at 115°F for a few minutes if it's solid)

¼ cup coconut nectar, raw honey, or raw agave nectar

1 teaspoon chili powder

½ teaspoon ground turmeric

1½ teaspoons coarse sea salt

4 green plantains

Plantains are starchy, particularly when they are in their green stage, making them less like a fruit and more like a potato. That makes them perfect chip material! They store for up to a month in an airtight container, so you might want to double up on the recipe if you have the larger Excalibur model. The longer you dry them, the crisper they get; but if you're short on time, you can eat them while they are still chewy.

Cut the lime in half and squeeze the juice into a large bowl. Whisk in the oil, coconut nectar, chili powder, turmeric, and salt. Fill a separate large bowl with water and toss the squeezed lime halves into the water.

Using a mandoline or very sharp knife, slice the plantains into ⅛-inch-thick rounds. As you cut them, place the slices into the acidulated water. When you've sliced them all, drain them and pat dry. Add to the oil mixture and toss to coat.

Arrange the plantain slices on ParaFlexx-lined dehydrator trays (you'll need about 4 ParaFlexx sheets) and place in the dehydrator. Set the machine to 105°F and dehydrate for 12 hours. Turn the chips over and onto mesh screens and dehydrate for another 12 to 20 hours, until crisp.

zucchini chips

{ MAKES ABOUT 4 DEHYDRATOR TRAYS }

2 medium zucchini, trimmed

2 tablespoons cold-pressed extra-virgin olive oil

¼ to ½ teaspoon sea salt

1 teaspoon mixed dried herbs, such as rosemary, oregano, and thyme

Zucchini is a raw foodist's best friend. We turn it into noodles with abandon (and without guilt!) to satisfy the craving for pasta, and here it makes an appearance in chip form. Gone are the "just one more chip" days—these chips are so nutritious and delicious that you'll want to eat as many as possible!

Using a mandoline or very sharp knife, slice the zucchini into ⅛-inch-thick rounds. Place them in a bowl, add the oil, and toss to coat well. Add the salt and herbs and toss to coat. Arrange the slices in a single layer on 4 ParaFlexx-lined dehydrator trays. Place in the dehydrator, set it to 115°F, and dehydrate for about 6 hours. Turn the chips over onto mesh screens and dehydrate for about another 5 hours, until crisp. Store in an airtight container for up to 1 week.

light as a feather apple chips

{ **MAKES AS MANY AS YOU LIKE** }

½ lemon

Apples (you decide how many)

Ground cinnamon or nutmeg (optional)

To make these chips, the apples are cut so thin that there is no need to peel them or remove the core, and the seeds pop right out. The chips come out of the dehydrator a visually stunning cross-section of an apple, practically translucent, crisp, and ethereal.

Fill a bowl with cold water. Squeeze the lemon half into the bowl and toss in the lemon.

Remove the stems from the apples and, using a mandoline, cut the apples crosswise into ⅛-inch-thick slices. As you slice them, immediately toss them into the acidulated water. Drain the slices, pat them dry, and arrange them in a single layer on mesh screen–lined dehydrator trays. Sprinkle with cinnamon if you like. Place in the dehydrator, turn the machine to 115°F, and dehydrate for 12 hours. Turn the chips over and dehydrate for another 12 to 20 hours, until crisp. Store in an airtight container for up to 1 week.

sweet and sour kale chips

{ **MAKES ABOUT 3 DEHYDRATOR SHEETS** }

2 bunches kale

¼ cup cold-pressed extra-virgin olive oil

3 tablespoons raw apple cider vinegar

¼ cup raw agave nectar

¾ teaspoon sea salt

Kale is the unofficial state vegetable of Vermont, according to my coauthor, Leda Scheintaub, who lives in the Green Mountain State. Vermonters certainly know what wholesome food is, and they can't get enough of this nutrient-rich, fiber-filled cruciferous vegetable. It seems every gardener grows a patch, and it is served up in a host of different ways.

Try this untraditional recipe, even if you think you don't like kale—it just might get you to change your mind. I've noticed that oven-roasted kale chips have come onto the culinary scene lately and have created something of a buzz. Kale chips made in the dehydrator are even better, though, as, of course, they are raw, but also because they "cook" more evenly—they come out uniformly crisp, and there's no watching over an oven to avoid burning!

You can use curly kale or the flat kind, known as dinosaur or lacinato kale. If you use curly kale, you'll need to leave space between the dehydrator trays, as the kale has some height to it. It will shrink considerably as it dehydrates. This is a relative quickie for a dehydrator recipe—just 4 to 6 hours in the machine.

Remove the stems from the kale, and then wash the leaves and dry thoroughly. Tear into bite-size pieces and place in a large bowl.

In a small bowl, whisk together the oil, vinegar, agave, and salt. Add it to the kale and stir to coat, then massage the marinade in for a couple of minutes to coat it thoroughly.

Place on ParaFlexx-lined dehydrator trays and place in the dehydrator. Set the machine to 115°F and dehydrate for 4 to 6 hours, until crisp. Eat immediately or store in an airtight container, where the chips will keep for up to 1 week.

fruit or vegetable leather

Fruits or vegetables

Lemon juice or sweetener (optional)

Fresh herbs or seasonings (optional)

Take them anywhere, roll 'em up! They are easy to carry and they are one of the simplest recipes in the book: all you need is fruits or vegetables and you're just about there. The type and amount of fruit or vegetable is entirely up to you. Feel free to add a touch of lemon juice, some herbs or other seasonings, or a little sweetener if you are dehydrating tart fruits such as cranberries.

A few suggestions: mango and cilantro, cranberry and mint, pineapple and salt, tomatoes and chili powder, pumpkin and nutmeg, peas and horseradish.

Use kitchen scissors to cut the leather into strips; roll it up to make your own fruit roll-ups—great for your kids' lunchboxes.

Cut the fruit or vegetables into chunks, place in a blender, and blend until smooth, adding a little water if necessary to get things moving.

Evenly spread the mixture onto ParaFlexx-lined dehydrator trays about ¼ inch thick. Place in the dehydrator, turn the machine to 115°F, and dehydrate for 8 to 12 hours. Flip over onto the mesh screen and dehydrate for another 8 to 12 hours until dry but malleable. Cut into strips.

menu ideas

SUNDAY BRUNCH BUFFET

- Tomato Ice Water
- Gravlax with Must-Have Mustard and Old World Cucumber Pickles
- Just Bananas Pancakes with Applesauce
- Triple Orange Salad with Pistachios and Mint or any fresh fruit salad

LUNCHBOX SELECTIONS

- Nutty Butter and jam on Lemon Bread
- Prosciutto or bresaola with Must-Have Mustard on Onion Caraway Flatbread
- Creamy Red Bell Pepper Dip with tomatoes and sprouts on Live Sun-Dried Tomato Bread
- Room for 'Shrooms and Walnut Pâté with cucumber slices on Garlicky Vegetable Flax Crackers

AFTERNOON TEA AND SWEETS

- A selection of warm teas
- Ginger Ale
- Hibiscus Lemonade
- Flax Crackers topped with Okima's Nori Cheese and Gravlax
- Goin' on a Date Rolls
- Lemon "Luv" Cupcakes with Coconut Meringue

PAN-ASIAN

- Salty Cucumber and Wakame Salad
- Gingery Squash and Coconut Noodle Soup and/or Thai-Style Mango Salad
- Chinese Broccoli in Garlic Soy Sauce
- Tuna Rolls with Ponzu Sauce and Spicy Mayonnaise

INDIAN STREET FOOD

- Rosewater, Salt, or Mango Lassi
- Indian-Style Papaya Salad
- Beets and Carrots with Coconut
- Chat

CRUDO MEXICANO

- Watermelon Agua Fresca or Tamarind Water
- Mexican Layered Salad
- Pico de Gallo
- Cumin-Corn-Cacao Crackers
- Maya Chocolate Pie

AN ALL-AMERICAN MEAL

- Green salad with Down on the Ranch Dressing
- Abundance Burgers with Marinated Mushrooms and Jícama Fries
- One Lucky Duck's Raw Ice Cream or Rum Raisin Ice Cream

DINNER IN UNDER AN HOUR

- Romaine lettuce salad with Easiest Umeboshi Vinaigrette
- Pasta with Tomato Sauce
- "Soft Serve" Frozen Fruit

SEXY, SOPHISTICATED DINNER

- Cantaloupe and Pomegranate Soup
- Fennel and Radicchio Salad with Raspberry Vinaigrette
- Lapsang Souchong Wild Mushrooms with Fresh Corn Polenta
- Frozen Chocolate Truffles

MOVIE NIGHT SNACKS

- "Popcorn" Cauliflower Crunchies
- Garlicky Salt and Vinegar Potato Chips
- Flax Crackers with Creamy Red Bell Pepper Dip
- Chocolate Chocolate Chip Cookies

swapping list

Time to turn your food world upside down—and have some fun while we're at it! As I've mentioned, there are a whole lot more raw offerings to choose from than when I first began my journey, and here I'm going to share some of my favorites. This list takes some of our top must-have foods—from banana bread to veggie burgers—and sets you up with their raw twin. And if you're a chocoholic, you will have choices aplenty, from chocolate syrup to peanut butter cups. Go to the individual manufacturers' Web sites (see Sources, page 239) to find even more flavors and varieties.

Keep in mind that not everyone will like every raw food—just as no one likes every cooked food. Figuring out your preferences may take some trial and error, so I encourage you to start with an open mind and a sense of playfulness. Once you know what your choices are, your default food options will change, and staying raw will become easy, just like I promised it would be!

BANANA BREAD

- Good Stuff by Mom & Me Banana Bread

BLONDIES

- Aimee's Livin' Magic Wild Vanilla Blondies

BREAD

- Aimee's Livin' Magic Herbed Onion Bread
- Good Stuff by Mom & Me's Tastes Like Rye
- Raw Girl Organic Sun-Flax Rye Bread
- Love Force Sun Bread (Flax, Focaccia, Italian, Raisin, Rye)
- Lydia's Organics Sunflower Seed Bread
- Raw Makery Bread (Garlic, Herb, Rye)

BREADSTICKS

- Raw Makery Bread Stix (Curry, Garlic, Rye)

BREAKFAST CEREALS

- Aimee's Livin' Magic SuperHero Cereal, Sprouted Granola
- Earthling Organics Rawnola (Cacao, Vanilla Bean)
- Emmy's Organics Almond Granola
- Good Stuff by Mom & Me Granola (Classic, Walnut Ginger Zinger, Sweet Almond), Buckwheaties, Muesli
- Go Raw Live Granola (Apple, Sprouted Cinnamon Chocolate, Simple)

- Lydia's Organics Grainless Cereals (Apple, Apricot, Berry, Sprouted Cinnamon, Vanilla)
- One Lucky Duck Crunchies (Chocolate, Cinnamon)
- Two Moms in the Raw Granola (Almond Butter Cacao Truffle, Blueberry, Cranberry, Gojiberry, and Raisin)

BREAKFAST (OR PROTEIN) DRINK

- Rockin' Wellness Nutritional Shake

BROWNIES

- Aimee's Livin' the Good Life Brownies
- Good Stuff by Mom & Me Brownies (Cacao Crackle Crunch, Walnut Fudge)

CARROT CAKE

- Good Stuff by Mom & Me Carrot Cake Loaf

CHEESECAKE

- Awesome Foods Raw Cheeze Cake (Blueberry, Chocolate, Plain)
- Organic Avenue Vegan New York–Style Cheesecake

CHIPS

- Aimee's Livin' Magic Hot Mama's Zucchini Chips
- Alive and Radiant Foods Kale Chips
- Brad's Raw Chips (Beet, Cheddar, Indian, Kale, Naked, Nasty Hot, Red Bell Pepper, Sun Dried Tomato, Sweet Potato, Vampire Killer)
- Love Force Kale Chips
- Lydia's Organics Kale Krunchies
- Nutritious Creations Sour Cream and Onion Kale Chips

CHOCOLATE BARS

- Gnosis Chocolate Bars
- Lydia's Organics Cacao Crunch Bars
- One Lucky Duck Chocolate Bars

- Organic Nectars Raw Cacao Chocolate Bar
- Righteously Raw 90% Cacao Bar with Caramel
- Xoçai Chocolate Nuggets and Squares

CHOCOLATE EASTER EGGS

- Aimee's Livin' Magic Golden Chocolate Eggs

CHOCOLATE HEARTS

- Sacred Chocolate Sacred Hearts (Coco Nibby, White Passion, Immuno Mushroom)

CHOCOLATE NUT BUTTER

- Rawtella Chocolate Hazelnut Spread

CHOCOLATE SYRUP

- Emmy's Organics Chocolate Sauce and Peppermint Chocolate Sauce
- Organic Nectars Organic Chocolate Dessert Syrup (also in Vanilla)

CHOCOLATE TRUFFLES

- ChocAlive! Chocolate Truffles

- Go Raw Chocolate Truffles
- Sacred Chocolate Sacred Truth (many flavors) Truffles

COOKIES

- Alive and Radiant Foods Raweos Sandwich Cookies (Chai, Fudge, Lemon)
- Emmy's Organics Raw Macaroons (Coconut-Vanilla, Dark Cacao, Lemon-Ginger, Mint Chip, Vegan Chai Spice)
- Go Raw Chocolate Cookies
- One Lucky Duck Cookies (Chocolate Chip, Macaroons, Raspberry Thumbprint)
- Organic Avenue Chocolate Macaroons

CRACKERS

- Aimee's Livin' Magic Crackers (Apple Cinnamon, Curry 'Kraut Chia, Dill Kimchee, Sun-dried Tomato)
- Go Raw Flax Crackers (Pizza, Simple, Sunflower)
- Lydia's Organics Crackers (Ginger-Nori, Green, Italian)

(continued)

swapping list (continued)

- Organic Avenue Crackers (Carrot Flax, Chia Flax, Veggie Seed)

DONUTS

- Good Stuff by Mom & Me Donut Holes (Apple Cinnamon, Cacao-Coconut, Gingerbread, Hazelnut Orange Chip, Lemon Chia)

FIG BARS

- Good Stuff by Mom & Me Fig Bars

FREEZE-DRIED FRUITS AND VEGETABLES

- Just Tomatoes

FRUIT LEATHER

- Kaia Foods Fruit Leather (Goji Orange, Lime Ginger, Spiced Apple, Vanilla Pear)

FUDGE

- Awesome Foods Fudge (Almond Butter, Carob Coconut, Chocolate, Chocolate Mint, Coconut Goji, Vanilla Mesquite Coconut)

GINGERBREAD

- Good Stuff by Mom & Me Ginger Bread

GINGER SNAPS

- Go Raw Ginger Snaps

GRANOLA BARS/ENERGY BARS

- Go Raw Live Granola Bars and Energy Bars
- Live Live & Organic Energy Bars (Oat Vanilla Goji)
- Love Force Energy Bars
- Rawnola Bars (Cacao, Vanilla Bean)
- Raw Revolution Live Food Bars and Green Bars (many flavors)
- Wildbar Meal in a Bar (Mayan Spice, Mountain Mint)

HOT SAUCE

- Real Pickles Tomatillo Hot Sauce

ICE CREAM

- One Lucky Duck Ice Cream
- Organic Nectars Cashewtopia Gelato

INSTANT SOUP

- Quantum Nutrition Tomato Soup Concentrate

JUICE IN THE BOTTLE

- Harmless Harvest raw coconut water
- Zukay Live Foods Kvass (Beet, Beet Ginger, Carrot Ginger, Veggie Medley)

MISO

- Miso Master Organic Miso
- South River Miso

NOODLES

- Sea Tangle Kelp Noodles

NUT BRITTLE

- Didi's Baking for Health Better Than Brittle
- Good Stuff by Mom & Me Caramelized Nut Mix

NUT BUTTERS

- Better Than Roasted Nut Butters
- Love Raw Foods Raw Nut Butters
- Rejuvenative Foods Nut and Seed Butters

ONION CRISPS

- Aimee's Livin' Magic Onion Crisps

PEANUT BUTTER CUPS

- Aimee's Livin' Magic Peanut Butter Cups

PECAN PIE

- Good Stuff by Mom and Me Pecan Pie Bars

PICKLES AND RELISH

- Bubbies Pure Kosher Dill Pickles and Dill Relish
- Real Pickles Dill Pickles, Garlic Dill Pickles, and Spicy Dill Pickles
- Zukay Live Foods Relish (Garlic Dill, Horseradish Dill)

SALAD DRESSING

- Zukay Live Foods Salad Dressing (Carrot Ginger, Cucumber Mint, Red Pepper Cilantro, Sweet Onion Basil, Tomato Pepper Pesto, Tomato Provençal)

SALSA

- Zukay Live Foods Salsa (Mild or Hot)

SAUERKRAUT

- Cultured Organic Pickle Shop Sauerkraut (many varieties)
- Real Pickles Sauerkraut (Plain, Garlic Kraut, Red Cabbage)

SOY SAUCE

- Nama Shoyu from Ohsawa

ARTIFICIAL SWEETENER

- Stevia (from natural foods stores)

TORTILLAS/WRAPS

- Pure Wraps Coconut Wraps
- Raw Makery Rawtillas

TRAIL MIX

- Aimee's Livin' Magic SuperHero Galactic Trail Mix
- Go Raw Sprouted Seed Mixes
- Living Intentions Gone Nuts!
- Lydia's Organics Savory Trail Mix
- Sunfood Nature's Abundance Snack Mix

VEGGIE BURGERS

- Awesome Foods Veggie Burgers

thank you

To Dr. Timothy Brantley: for all the hours spent on the phone with me making sure I was expressing myself correctly. I don't have enough words of gratitude! You are where it all started for me. You are a genius, a pioneer, a generous person, and a great and loving friend.

Dr. Nicholas Gonzalez: for keeping me healthy, always supporting me, and answering all my questions—I think you are amazing.

Christopher Dobrowolski: my friend, my inspiration, and my last-minute ace in the hole. I just adore you!

Dr. Richard Firshein: for jumping on board with your thoughts, help, and enthusiasm.

Udo Erasmus: for your expertise on oils and fats, and for making your wonderful oil and your wonderful daughter, Usha.

Usha Menard: for the cover and interior photos—they're great! And for your constant support.

Patty White: for your wonderful food styling for the cover and interior photos and long hours of work! The pictures (at the risk of repeating myself) are fabulous.

Sae Ryun Song: for cover makeup, and Tatiana Boyko, for cover hair—brilliant work!

To our talented and generous recipe contributors—what an honor: Marilyn Chiarello, Christopher Dobrowolski, Michael Durr, Doug Evans, Kieba, Claire Lunny, Sarma Melngailis, Leah Mutz, Nash Patel, Marie Pavillard, Tanya Petrich, Ani Phyo, RawChefDan, Cherie Soria, Terry Walters, Okima Wilcox-Hitt, and Tatiana Yashin.

Laura Dail: my agent, my friend, and my inspiration.

My mom, Muriel, and my sisters, Christine Gnatowsky and Karen Roos: for the lively conversation and support in all I do.

Aliza Fogelson: you are the most amazing editor! I appreciate all your scrutiny and creativity. This would be half the book it is without you.

Jane Treuhaft: for your creativity and sensitivity to our desires at the photo shoot.

To my team at Clarkson Potter: publisher Lauren Shakely, editorial director Doris Cooper, production editor Tricia Wygal, production manager Joan Denman, designer Rae Ann Spitzenberger, as well as assistant editor Ashley Phillips: without you this book would not be as fabulous, would not look as wonderful. You all added to this experience. Thank you!

Liana Krissoff: for your insightful review of our writing. And Deborah Kops for her excellent copyediting.

Leda Scheintaub: words cannot express . . . the process was incredible. Your willingness to learn, your enthusiasm, your spirit. I would do it again . . .

Alexei Yashin: mon amour.

sources

Consider this a jumping-off point to get you started on your raw journey. This is my personal list, but I'm sure you'll find some more great resources along the way that you won't be able to live without. Just look, all you couch potatoes (like me!), it's easy to click on the computer and get fabulous raw food delivered!

AIMEE'S LIVIN' MAGIC
www.aimeeslivinmagic.com
207-409-0899
Breakfast cereal, blondies, brownies, chocolate bars, chocolate eggs, crackers, dried fruit, nuts and seeds, onion bread, onion crisps, peanut butter cups, peppermint swirls, salt, trail mix, zucchini chips

ALIVE AND RADIANT FOODS
www.blessingsaliveandradiantfoods.com
Raweos (sandwich cookies), kale chips

AWESOME FOODS
www.awesomefoods.com
610-757-1048
Bars, breads, cheesecake, cookies, dressings, fudge, onion rings, vegetable chips, veggie burgers

BINESHII WILD RICE
www.bineshiiwildrice.com
800-484-2347
Truly raw wild rice

BLUE MOUNTAIN ORGANICS
www.bluemountainorganics.com
866-777-7475
Better Than Roasted sprouted nut and seed butters

BODY ECOLOGY DIET
www.bodyecology.com
800-511-2660
Kefir starter, stevia concentrate

BRAD'S RAW FOODS
www.bradsrawchips.com
215-766-3739
Vegetable chips in many varieties

BRANTLEY LIVING HERBAL FORMULAS
www.brantleycure.com
Digestive enzymes, nutritional supplements, and other products

BUBBIES
www.bubbies.com
Pickles and relish
(Available in the refrigerated section of natural foods stores)

CAMPAIGN FOR REAL MILK
www.realmilk.com
State-by-state listing of farms that sell raw milk

CHOCALIVE!
www.chocalive.com
877-246-2254
Chocolate truffles

COCONUT SECRETS
www.coconutsecret.com
888-369-3393
Coconut aminos, coconut crystals, coconut flour, coconut nectar, coconut vinegar
(Products also available in many natural foods stores)

CULTURED PICKLE SHOP
www.culturedpickleshop.com
510-540-5185
Pickled vegetables, kim chee, and sauerkraut
(Retail store in Berkeley, CA)

DIDI'S BAKING FOR HEALTH
www.bakingforhealth.com
212-505-2232
Breakfast cereals, nut brittle, pies, snacks

EARTHLING ORGANICS
www.earthlingorganics.com
760-289-5188
Rawnola, Rawnola bars

EARTHSOURCE ORGANICS
www.earthsourceorganics.com
760-510-1561
Righteously Raw chocolate bars,
chocolate with caramel bars

EATWILD
www.eatwild.com
State-by-state directory of farms that sell
local grass-fed meat, eggs, and dairy

EMMY'S ORGANICS
www.emmysorganics.foodzie.com
Chocolate sauce, granola, macaroons

EXCALIBUR
www.excaliburdehydrator.com
800-875-4254
Dehydrators

**FARM-TO-CONSUMER LEGAL DEFENSE
FUND**
www.farmtoconsumer.org
State-by-state review of raw milk laws

FOOD FOR LIFE
Ezekiel sprouted bread, English muffins,
tortillas, buns, pasta, wraps (bridge food:
cooked but sprouted)
(Available in many natural foods stores in
the frozen foods section)

GEM CULTURES
www.gemcultures.com
253-588-2922
Kefir starter

GNOSIS CHOCOLATE
www.gnosischocolate.com
646-688-5549
Chocolate bars

GOLD MINE NATURAL FOOD CO.
www.goldminenaturalfoods.com
800-475-3663
Kelp noodles, miso, Ohsawa nama shoyu,
sea vegetables, umeboshi plums and
vinegar

GOOD STUFF BY MOM & ME
www.gimmegoodstuff.com
888-797-6865
Almond bars, banana bread, brownies,
carrot cake, caramelized nut mix, coconut
nectar and vinegar, donut holes, ginger
bread, granola, muesli, nuts and seeds,
olives, pecan pie bars, rye bread, sea salt,
sprouters

GO RAW
www.goraw.com
650-962-9299
Bars, chocolate, chocolate truffles, chips,
crackers, cookies, energy bars, ginger
snaps granola, granola bars, green bars,
sprouted seeds
(Also available in many natural foods
stores)

GREAT EASTERN SUN
www.great-eastern-sun.com
800-334-5809
Organic miso, sea vegetables

GRILLO'S PICKLES
www.grillospickles.com
860-884-4382
Natural pickles
(Available at stores in Connecticut,
Maine, Massachusetts, New York, and
Rhode Island)

HARMLESS HARVEST
www.harmlesscoconut.com
347-688-6286
Raw coconut water
(Also available in some natural foods
stores)

JUST TOMATOES ETC!
www.justtomatoes.com
800-537-1985
Freeze-dried fruit and vegetable snacks

KAIA FOODS
www.kaiafoods.com
510-238-0128
Breakfast cereals, fruit leather,
sprouted nuts

KEVITA PROBIOTIC DRINKS
kevita.com
888-310-6106
Vegan probiotic superdrink made
with kefir

LIVE LIVE & ORGANIC
www.live-live.com
877-505-5504/212-505-5504
Comprehensive shopping site: Appliances
(blenders, dehydrators, juicers, nut milk
bags, spiral slicers, sprouters), body-
care products, books and DVDs, breads,
breakfast cereals, brownies, chocolate,
coconut products, crackers, dried fruit,
energy bars, green powders, ice cream,
kelp noodles, lucuma powder, nuts and

seeds, nut and seed butters, nut mixes,
oils, olives, sandwich cookies, sea salt,
sea vegetables, snacks, sprouting seeds,
sweeteners, vegetable chips
(Retail store in New York City)

LIVING INTENTIONS
www.shop.livingintentions.com
Gone Nuts! nut mixes

LOCAL HARVEST
www.localharvest.org
Directory of farmers' markets, family
farms, and other sources of sustainably
grown food in your area, including
restaurants, natural foods stores, and
co-ops

LOVE FORCE
www.loveforce.net
513-470-1787
Breads, energy bars, kale chips

LYDIA'S ORGANICS
www.lydiasorganics.com
415-258-9678
Breads, cereals, chips, chocolate bars,
crackers, energy bars, green powder,
kale chips, trail mix

MAGIC BULLET
www.buythebullet.com
866-446-6352
Blenders

MANNA ORGANICS
www.mannaorganicbakery.com
Sprouted breads (a bridge food: cooked
on the outside, raw on the inside;
available in many natural foods stores
in the frozen foods section)

MEDICINE FLOWER
www.medicineflower.com
800-787-3645
Flavor extracts (including cherry, chocolate, coconut, mint, rum, strawberry, vanilla)

NUTRITIOUS CREATIONS
www.SmartSnacks.com
631-666-9815
Kale chips and other vegetable chips

ONE LUCKY DUCK
www.oneluckyduck.com
866-205-4895
Bars, breakfast cereals, chocolate bars, chocolate truffles, coconut oil, cookies, dried fruit, ice cream, lucuma powder, nuts and seeds, nut and seed butters, nutritional yeast, sea salt, sea vegetables, stevia, sweeteners, oils
(Retail store in New York City)

ORGANIC AVENUE
www.organicavenue.com
212-358-0500
Comprehensive shopping site: Appliances (blenders, dehydrators, juicers, nut milk bags, spiral slicers, sprouters), books and DVDs, breakfast cereal, breads, cheesecake, chips, chocolate bars, chocolate truffles, chocolate and vanilla sauce, coconut oil, cookies, crackers, dips, donut holes, dried fruit, juices, kelp noodles, lucuma powder, nuts and seeds, nut and seed butters, nut mixes, oils, Rawnola, salt, sea vegetables, snack bars, sweeteners, vegan cheeses
(Retail stores in New York City)

ORGANIC NECTARS
www.organicnectars.com
845-246-0506
Agave, agave dessert syrups (chocolate and vanilla), agave syrup, cacao, Cashewtopia gelato, chocolate bars, goji berries, PalmSweet powdered coconut sugar

PH ION
www.ph-ion.com
888-744-8589
Mineral powder and greens

PHRESH GREENS
www.phreshgreens.me
302-357-9611
Powdered greens

PURE WRAPS
www.thepurewraps.com
404-585-7873
Wraps made from coconut meat

QUANTUM NUTRITION LABS
www.quantumnutrition.com
800-325-7734
Nutritional yeast, tomato soup concentrate

RAW FOOD WORLD STORE
www.therawfoodworld.com
866-729-3438
Comprehensive shopping site: Appliances (blenders, dehydrators, juicers, nut milk bags, spiral slicers, sprouters), bulk raw foods, cacao powder, chocolate bars, coconut products, dried fruit, flavor extracts, grains, green powders, herbs, ice cream, kelp noodles, nama shoyu, nuts and seeds, nut and seed butters, olives, oils, sea vegetables, snacks, sprouting seeds, yacon syrup and other sweeteners

RAWGURU
www.rawguru.com
800-577-4729
Comprehensive shopping site: Appliances (blenders, dehydrators, juicers, nut milk bags, spiral slicers, sprouters, sushi mats), cacao, cereals, chocolate, condiments and seasonings, cookies, crackers, dried fruits, grains, ice cream, oils, olives, nuts and seeds, nut and seed butters, sandwich cookies, sea salt, sea vegetables, snacks, sprouting seeds, sweeteners, vegetable chips, young coconuts

RAW MAKERY
www.rawmakery.com
Breads, breadsticks, cookies, crackers, krispies, rawtillas

RAW REVOLUTION
www.rawrev.com
866-498-4671
Live food bars and green superfood bars

RAWTELLA
www.rawtella.com
800-577-4729
Rawtella chocolate hazelnut spread

RAWVOLUTION
Rawvolution.com
800-9976-RAW
Matt Amsden's weekly food menus delivered anywhere in the United States

REAL PICKLES
www.realpickles.com
413-774-2600
Pickles, pickled beets, sauerkraut, tomatillo hot sauce
(Available at stores in the Northeast)

REJUVENATIVE FOODS
www.rejuvenative.com
800-805-7957
Raw nut and seed butters

ROCKIN' WELLNESS
rockinwellness.com
855-UROCKWELL
Raw nutrition shake mix

SACRED CHOCOLATE
www.sacredchocolate.com
415-456-3311
Chocolate bars, chocolate hearts, chocolate truffles, nut and seed butters

SEA TANGLE NOODLE COMPANY
www.kelpnoodles.com
408-966-3109
Kelp noodles

SHOP RAW FOODS
www.shoprawfoods.com
Comprehensive shopping site: Breads, condiments, cookies, crackers, chips, chocolate, coconut products, dried fruits, energy bars, kelp noodles, nuts and seeds, nut and seed butters, nut milk bags, oils, olives, sea vegetables, stevia, spices, sprouting seeds, yacon syrup and other sweeteners

SOUTH RIVER MISO
www.southrivermiso.com
413-369-4057
Naturally aged miso

SUNFOOD
www.sunfood.com
888-729-3663
Comprehensive shopping site: Appliances (blenders, dehydrators, juicers, spiral slicers, sprouters), breakfast cereals, cacao butter and powder, chocolate bars, chocolate hearts, chocolate truffles, coconut oil, dried fruit, energy bars, green superfood supplements, herbs and spices, nuts and seeds, oils, olives, sea vegetables, snacks, sprouting seeds, sweeteners, trail mix, wraps

TWO MOMS IN THE RAW
www.twomomsintheraw.com
720-221-8555
Raw granolas and bars

UBRAW
www.ubraw.com
702-346-5029
Coconut noodler

U.S. WELLNESS MEATS
www.uswellnessmeats.com
877-383-0051
Humanely raised meats

VITAMIX
www.vitamix.com
800-848-2649
High-speed blender

VIVAPURA
www.vivapura.net
877-787-6457
Comprehensive shopping site: almonds and other nuts, breads, cacao powder, coconut products, cereals, chips, crackers, dried fruits, grains, lucuma powder, nut and seed butters, nutritional yeast, snacks, oils, olives, sea vegetables, sweeteners, trail mix

WILDBAR
www.wildbar.info
Meal in a bar

YÓGOURMET
www.lyo-san.ca
450-562-8525
Kefir starter
(Also available in some natural foods stores, including Whole Foods)

XOÇAI
www.thehealthychocolate.com
866-219-9067
Chocolate nuggets and squares, fortified with omega-3 fatty acids, probiotics, and/ or flax seeds

ZUKAY LIVE FOODS
www.zukay.com
610-286-3077
Dressings, relishes, salsas, vegetable juices
(Available in many natural foods stores)

appendix: in my opinion . . . what it means to be raw

Let me state the obvious here: I am neither a doctor nor a scientist. I'm a model and an actress, and I prefer to write in language that normal, everyday people can understand. So, let me tell you—in layman's terms, in my own words—what I believe really happens to food when you cook it. There are four important concerns:

1. The molecular structure changes.

2. The pH could be affected.

3. Enzymes are destroyed.

4. The bonds between vitamins and minerals break down.

Let's look more closely at each of these:

1. The Molecular Structure Changes.

Changing the molecular structure of your food—cooking it—is a big mess. But, you protest, you like your veg- etables cooked because they taste better. I hear you, but you should know that the difference between a raw and a cooked vegetable is literally the differ- ence between life and death. Really, I'm not trying to be a drama queen here— well, yes, maybe I am! But I did get your attention, didn't I?

Let me try to explain. I took high school chemistry. OK, I barely passed high school chemistry. Thankfully the teacher liked me or I probably would have failed. I didn't see how chemistry pertained to the real world or my everyday life. I remember taking two clear liquids and mixing them, and then taking the clear liquid mixture that resulted and adding heat. Voilà— it changed color! Big deal, I thought.

It actually is a big deal, and years later when I went raw, it suddenly made sense. If you add heat, the molecular structure changes (indicated by the color change of the liquid in the case of my chemistry class experiment). So then I wondered, does the same thing happen when you cook food?

Well, Christopher Dobrowolski, the founder of Live Live & Organic, a raw foods market and resource center based in New York City, told me about some of the chemicals that are present in heated foods but not in raw, which led me to conclude that cooking causes problematic changes in food. Here are two examples.

First, high levels of PAHs (poly- aromatic hydrocarbons), by-products of fuel burning, are found in many cooked foods—for example, in meat cooked at high temperatures, such as grilling, and in smoked fish. PAHs are of concern because some of these compounds have been identified as carcinogenic.

Second, much of the food we eat contains acrylamide, a chemical created by cooking food (a worldwide alert was issued in 2002, when scientists made an announcement to this effect). The chemical can cause gene mutations, leading to a range of cancers in rats. Acrylamide is a naturally occurring chemical compound found in many plant-based, high-carbohydrate foods after they are heated. It appears that the chemical, which is used in the treatment of sewage and waste and to manufacture certain chemicals, plastics, and dyes, is also a by-product of cooking food at high temperatures.

> Whatever heating does on a molecular level, all I really need to know is this: the more raw I eat, the easier it is to digest raw—and it makes me feel better. Period. No stomachaches, no heartburn. What a relief after years of popping antacids.

Cooked food brings to mind using heat to make objects bond together and become more solid and stronger, like a heat gun to cure glue or an instrument a dentist will use to bond fillings. It seems to be the opposite of making digestion and absorption "easy"!

What does all this mean to the body? Well, if the body is set up to read the molecular structure of food, and you change that molecular structure, the

WHAT COOKING AND GENETIC ENGINEERING HAVE IN COMMON

Proponents of genetic engineering—manipulating the genes in one living thing, usually a food, with genes from another—say it will make our food supply cheaper and better. But to me it's pretty freaky. For instance, they have crossed a tomato with a brook trout to make that tomato resistant to cold like the hearty trout. Now that's just weird.

This form of messing with Mother Nature is very new. It was introduced into our food system in 1994, and there have been no scientific studies on the long-term consequences of genetic engineering. So what does genetic engineering have in common with cooking? They both change the structure of food on a molecular level. And the really scary thing about genetic engineering is that the food is changed on a molecular level before it is even cooked.

My point is this: If you don't cook your food because it changes the molecular structure, then certainly you would want to stay clear of genetically engineered food. Please look for foods that are labeled 100% organic or GMO-free. Genetically modifying crops is big business—so favor small local farmers and farmers' markets to stay free of GMO foods.

saving seeds to save the world

Back in the 1800s we had more than seven thousand varieties of apples. Imagine that. Now there are only about three hundred. What's going on?

Seeds traditionally have been passed down from generation to generation, but now most crops are planted on industrial farms with mass-produced seeds, and those seeds are often genetically modified. Loss of variety is the result and crops disappear on a daily basis.

The good news: Way up near the North Pole, our civilization is being saved, seed by seed. It is a project called the Svalbard Global Seed Vault, in an Arctic island administered by Norway called Spitsbergen. There, deep inside the vault in millions of little envelopes, scientists are safeguarding seeds: a billion and a half of them. The structure, also known as the Doomsday Vault, is built right into the ice and is designed to last ten thousand years; it is virtually indestructible. And as if the Arctic chill weren't enough to preserve those seeds, it's air-conditioned to guarantee a freezing temperature for a long time!

The vault houses seeds from just about every country from all the world's crops. The goal is to preserve our civilization by preserving the foods that have been keeping us going since time immemorial. The "doomsday" part is that the seeds are being protected from climate change, natural disasters, and man-made catastrophes, such as nuclear war. But the truth is we're experiencing a doomsday right now, as some plants are going extinct as a result of industrial farming and genetic engineering.

body has to change or work harder to get what nutrition it can out of that food.

And what does this do to the body? Well, since most scientists think that on an evolutionary level it takes about one million years for a species to fully adapt to an entirely new diet (pasteurized food has only been around since the beginning of the twentieth century), cooked, processed food might involve a much more drastic change than simply switching from one type of raw food to another, so it may take a much longer time to adjust to it. We may be able to tolerate it to some extent, but cooked doesn't seem to me to be the optimal choice.

2. The pH Changes.

Timothy Brantley, the doctor who introduced me to raw foods, and the author of the *New York Times* bestseller *The Cure: Heal Your Body, Save Your Life* (2007), taught me that the body needs to stay alkaline for health, but it creates all kinds of acid. That means almost anything we do—whether it's digesting food, working out, stressing out (and yes, even sex)—we are making acid. Our bodies make nothing alkaline. But our blood and fluids need to be in a slightly neutral to alkaline state, ideally between a pH of 7.42 and 7.36. How do we get there? One answer: Eat lots of raw food—especially veggies!

Throw acid on a car, and it will eat the paint away and go through the metal; likewise acid blood running through your system will go through your organs and wear your body down.

The connection between food and the acid/alkaline balance in the body is a most confusing subject (for example, lemons, which taste acidic, have an alkalizing effect on the body), and every expert has a different opinion. I've asked Christopher of Live Live & Organic to help us to better understand the concept. In his opinion, the only food category that is fully alkalizing (meaning it has an alkalizing effect on the body) is vegetables. Fruits are next, with a few exceptions. On the other hand, all meats and all dairy (except sour cream and maybe butter) are acidifying (meaning they have an acidifying effect on the body). All other groups of foods are a mixture. Beans are generally acidifying—adzuki, black, pinto, and kidney beans being the least acidifying. Most nuts and seeds are acidifying, with a few exceptions, including coconut, sesame seeds,

pumpkin seeds, and almonds. Most grains are acidifying, with the exception of quinoa, millet, and buckwheat (which technically is not a grain). Of course, these foods still have a lot of beneficial nutrients. The good news is that foods in their raw state generally are less acid forming than in their cooked state.

What you do with your food also has an effect on how acidifying it will be. Cooking destroys a lot of nutrients, disrupts the natural balance of biochemical elements, and makes food more acid. Another way to make your food easier to digest is to sprout—sprouting your nuts, seeds, grains, and beans will make them less acidic, more nutritious, and easier to digest.

I'll be the first to admit that I'm a type A personality—very acidic! But going from cooked to raw definitely mellowed me out a bit. Ask anyone: I still have my New York edge, but I don't get as hung up on the little things as I used to. This was a big help on Donald Trump's *Celebrity Apprentice*, when everyone tried to stress everyone else

STRESS≠SUCCESS

When I was modeling, I thought of my acid stomach as a badge of honor. I equated stress with success. But truthfully, I have just as much stress in my life now. The difference is that now my diet is no longer acidic, so I can handle the stress more easily. And no more acid stomach!

out so that they would lose their cool and make mistakes. I was so alkaline that they just couldn't get my goat! I noticed that when I went raw I became a whole lot less reactive right away. The more raw food I added to my diet, the less reactive I became and the better my decisions were.

So how do you know if you're acidic? Well, most of us are—more than half the population is hanging out in an acidic state. If you want to find out, buy some pH test strips (also called litmus paper)—you can find them in some health food stores or online. You can test and find out if your body is running acidic; the color of the strips will change and you'll compare it to the rainbow of colors on the box. Do this a few times throughout the day (not when you have just eaten, though) and average the numbers. By comparing the test strips with the box, you'll see if you're acidic or alkaline. If you're acidic, time to add raw. And time to consult with a doctor, as you should anytime you are thinking of making changes to your diet.

3. The Bonds Between Vitamins and Minerals and Proteins Change.

Sometimes change is a good thing, but not when you're talking vitamins and minerals. The bonds between the two are superfragile, and heat affects them immediately. While not all of the nutrients in food are destroyed by cooking, your body faces the Herculean task of trying to absorb nutrients when they are not in the natural state that it recognizes. Ask any woman who takes calcium; calcium supplements are best when they contain vitamin D and magnesium, because calcium can be absorbed more readily in the presence of vitamin D and magnesium, and vice versa. Cool, huh?

The best plan of action is to eat foods that are clean and that the body can recognize easily and utilize, and then get rid of what it doesn't need. And favor whole foods—the vitamins and minerals in the skin of an apple are as important for the absorption of nutrients as the vitamins and minerals in the meat of the apple. They work together to create a whole universe; your body recognizes it all and can utilize all of it.

4. Enzymes Are Destroyed.

We are born of an enzyme reaction, our lives are one big enzyme reaction, and when we die, an enzyme reaction breaks our bodies down into dust. Considering we're talking about life itself here, wouldn't you say we are just a bit cavalier when it comes to losing a few enzymes when we cook?

What are enzymes exactly? Enzymes are protein molecules that facilitate most of the body's metabolic processes, such as digestion. Health guru Dr. David Jubb would say that enzymes are little workers that act as catalysts and are needed for every single function of the body, from blinking an eye to digesting food. And of course there are metabolic enzymes and digestive enzymes supplying energy (hello—who couldn't use a little more energy, raise your hand!). There are literally thousands of metabolic and digestive enzymes; digestion alone can use up to 70 percent of the body's energy to break food down and get rid of waste.

Without enzymes, you can have a squeaky-clean diet and still feel less than healthy, because all that healthy food isn't being absorbed and used by your body. According to Dr. Edward Howell, a pioneer in the study of enzymes during the early part of the twentieth century and author of *Enzyme*

man, you killed it!

Enzymes are what make fruit ripen. When air hits the flesh of the fruit, the enzymes start to "digest" the fruit and the nutrients are released. This is when I want to eat it. The easier it is to get at the nutrients, the better it is for you. Nuts about nuts? A raw nut, like an almond for example, can germinate when soaked in water—which means it can start to grow and start releasing its nutrients. A cooked almond will not germinate—go figure. Heat causes so much of a chemical change that a cooked nut will never grow again. Same with legumes. Man, you killed it! I am a living being—why would I want to eat dead food?

Nutrition, we are given a finite amount of enzymes at birth. When they are gone, so are we.

Heat is the enemy of enzymes. So the best place to get enzymes is—you guessed it—raw food. This is where the magical raw temperature of 115°F comes from. Were you wondering? Anything heated above 115°F is pretty much dead or dying. Those digestive enzymes don't stand a chance! According to Dr. Howell, the body has to use up its own enzymes to help digest food—taking them away from other vital functions.

Raw foods naysayers will tell you that heating food isn't a big deal, that you may lose a few enzymes here and there when you cook, but that overall, cooked food is better for you because it's easier to digest. I can see why they think that: After a lifetime of cooked foods, your digestive enzymes are weaker and going raw may bother your stomach; it isn't sure what to think of this sudden change. Don't fret—there are tons of digestive enzymes available at your natural foods store or from your doctor (yes, you should always see a doctor when changing your diet). And adding a fresh-pressed juice or two to your menu will help get nutrition into your body more quickly.

In addition to dealing with weaker digestive enzymes, some people find vegetables (as well as nuts and seeds) hard to digest in the raw form, according to Christopher Dobrowolski of Live Live & Organic.

Besides weak enzymes, there are two other contributing factors:

1. A lack of good bacteria in the intestines. Sometimes just supplementing with probiotics or a pinch of Celtic sea salt before eating (most people's stomachs are underactive, and sea salt stimulates the production of hydrochloric acid in the stomach so you can better digest your food) or having an unpasteurized cultured beverage (like kombucha or a little juice from the bottom of a sauerkraut or pickle jar) can help!

2. A system that doesn't get cleaned of old gunk before eating new, clean food. But the good news is the more clean, healthy food you eat, the more optimally the system runs.

So with a little tweaking of your diet and the help of my recipes, Shopping List, Swapping List, and Sources, it's becoming easier to go raw in my book (pun intended!).

index